50 Studies Every Pediatrician Should Know

50 STUDIES EVERY DOCTOR SHOULD KNOW

Published and Forthcoming Books in the *50 Studies Every Doctor Should Know* Series

50 Studies Every Doctor Should Know: The Key Studies that Form the Foundation of Evidence Based Medicine, Revised Edition
Michael E. Hochman

50 Studies Every Internist Should Know
Edited by Kristopher Swiger, Joshua R. Thomas, Michael E. Hochman, and Steven D. Hochman

50 Studies Every Neurologist Should Know
Edited by David Y. Hwang and David M. Greer

50 Studies Every Surgeon Should Know
Edited by SreyRam Kuy and Rachel J. Kwon

50 Studies Every Pediatrician Should Know
Edited by Ashaunta T. Anderson, Nina L. Shapiro, Stephen C. Aronoff, Jeremiah Davis and Michael Levy

50 Imaging Studies Every Doctor Should Know
Christoph Lee

50 Studies Every Anesthesiologist Should Know
Anita Gupta

50 Studies Every Intensivist Should Know
Edward Bittner

50 Studies Every Psychiatrist Should Know
Vinod Srihari, Ish Bhalla, and Rajesh Tampi

50 Studies Every Pediatrician Should Know

ASHAUNTA T. ANDERSON, MD, MPH, MSHS
Assistant Professor of Pediatrics
University of California Riverside School of Medicine
Riverside, California
Health Policy Researcher
RAND Corporation
Santa Monica, California

NINA L. SHAPIRO, MD
Director of Pediatric Otolaryngology
Professor of Head and Neck Surgery
David Geffen School of Medicine
University of California Los Angeles
Los Angeles, California

STEPHEN C. ARONOFF, MD, MBA
Waldo E. Nelson Professor and
Chairperson, Department of Pediatrics
Lewis Katz School of Medicine
Temple University
Philadelphia, Pennsylvania

JEREMIAH C. DAVIS, MD, MPH
Community Pediatrician
Mosaic Medical
Bend, Oregon

MICHAEL LEVY, MD
Assistant Professor of Pediatrics and Communicable Diseases
University of Michigan
C.S. Mott Children's Hospital
Ann Arbor, Michigan

SERIES EDITOR:
MICHAEL E. HOCHMAN, MD, MPH
Assistant Professor of Clinical Medicine
Keck School of Medicine
University of Southern California
Los Angeles, California

OXFORD
UNIVERSITY PRESS

OXFORD
UNIVERSITY PRESS

Oxford University Press is a department of the University of Oxford. It furthers
the University's objective of excellence in research, scholarship, and education
by publishing worldwide. Oxford is a registered trade mark of Oxford University
Press in the UK and certain other countries.

Published in the United States of America by Oxford University Press
198 Madison Avenue, New York, NY 10016, United States of America.

© Oxford University Press 2016

First Edition published in 2016

Library of Congress Cataloging-in-Publication Data
Names: Anderson, Ashaunta T., editor. | Shapiro, Nina L., editor. | Aronoff,
Stephen C., editor. | Davis, Jeremiah, editor. | Levy, Michael, editor.
Title: 50 studies every pediatrician should know / [edited by] Ashaunta T. Anderson,
Nina L. Shapiro, Stephen C. Aronoff, Jeremiah Davis, and Michael Levy.
Other titles: Fifty studies every pediatrician should know | 50 studies every
doctor should know (Series)
Description: Oxford ; New York : Oxford University Press, [2016] | Series: 50
studies every doctor should know | Includes bibliographical references.
Identifiers: LCCN 2015039268 | ISBN 9780190204037 (alk. paper)
Subjects: | MESH: Pediatrics—methods. | Clinical Trials as Topic. |
Evidence-Based Medicine.
Classification: LCC RJ48 | NLM WS 200 | DDC 618.92—dc23
LC record available at http://lccn.loc.gov/2015039268

9 8 7 6 5 4 3
Printed by Webcom, Canada

For my son, Avery, and all the children we serve. I loved you before you were.

*For my mother, Ingrid, and husband, Anton, who taught me
the power of words and of love.*
— ASHAUNTA ANDERSON

For my family. And for my patients, who always teach me something.
— NINA SHAPIRO

*To the patients who allowed me to treat them and, in the end,
proved to be my best teachers.*
— STEPHEN ARONOFF

*To the patients I've yet to treat—may the knowledge herein help me
rise to the task.*
— JEREMIAH DAVIS

For Jen and Dad, the best pediatricians I know.
— MICHAEL LEVY

CONTENTS

PREFACE

At the turn of the last century, William Osler, the father of modern medicine and pediatrics, noted that the practice of medicine is "an art based on science." The science, in the late 1890s and early twentieth century, consisted mostly of anatomy, histology, pathology, and rudimentary microbiology. The medical literature of the day consisted of anecdotal observations and logical, well-reasoned treatises. Much of the knowledge of medicine was passed from master to apprentice and was largely dogmatic in nature.

Beginning in the late 1940s, medical evidence, as we have come to know it, was born. Beginning with the early trials of streptomycin therapy for tuberculosis and the Framingham Heart Study in the 1940s, the observations of Rammelcamp and Jones linking streptococcal pharyngitis and rheumatic fever, and the Salk polio vaccine trials in the 1950s, the amount of usable, scientifically based, medical evidence has grown at logarithmic rates. If Osler were alive today, he would probably state that the science of modern medicine, while inherently uncertain, is empiric and based on evidence generated by well-defined, rigorous methodologies. Unlike the generations of physicians who have gone before, today's medical practitioners have a wealth of evidence to use as touchstones in all aspects of medical decision-making, enabling all of us to practice a higher quality of medicine and to ensure that, above all else, we do no harm.

This book and the other volumes in the Oxford University Press series, *50 Studies Every Doctor Should Know*, represent the cumulative "canon" that many physicians have created individually and together to try to better understand the evidence behind our practice. With the rapid increase in scientific literature publishing over the past two decades, selecting only 50 titles to include may seem unnecessarily restrictive. Our goal with this first edition was to uncover the original studies that inform key areas of pediatric medical decision making, recognizing that this evidence is imperfect and inherently uncertain.

Nevertheless, the studies presented in this volume are, as best we can determine, the controlling evidence at this point in time.

The process of identifying the studies included: (1) recruitment of authors around the United States in both academic and community settings, in general pediatrics and subspecialty pediatrics; and (2) the development of a preliminary list of those studies we felt were most important to how pediatrics is currently practiced. This list was shared with national experts in pediatrics in an effort to include the most pivotal studies available. The final list of candidate articles was divided among team members and each article was summarized; these summaries were shared with original authors whenever possible for feedback, comment, and correction. When original authors were unavailable, members of their research teams were solicited, and, if needed, national experts in the appropriate subspecialties were consulted. We are incredibly fortunate to have had so many original authors discuss their work with us and, through this collaboration, make our summaries more accurate and reflective of the original works' intention.

Perhaps more than any other area of medicine, pediatrics struggles to amass a sufficient evidence base for many of our interventions. Studies involving children are inherently more circumspect with regard to consent, risk, and determining long-term benefit. Many pediatric illnesses are rare, making significant conclusions difficult to come by at single centers. Whenever possible, we tried to seek "gold standard" study designs such as randomized, placebo-controlled, double-blind investigations. Admittedly, there are a fair number of studies included in this volume that fall short of what is today considered the gold standard for medical evidence. Our team made a conscious decision to include many of these trials simply because they continue to underpin pediatric medicine. It is our hope that an in-depth examination of these classic articles will provide the reader with a better understanding of the uncertainty and limitations of the evidence commonly used in medical decision making, allowing the reader to make more informed choices for their own patients. To help this effort, each article summary includes discussion of related articles—many of which are more current and often explain how our thinking as pediatricians has changed with better-designed studies in more recent publications. We also include a relevant case presentation at the conclusion of each chapter, to better illustrate the clinical relevance of each article.

Hopefully this collection of pediatric articles adds new insight into your practice, reveals some publications that may not have been part of your own canon, and fosters discussions of what evidence we all should be using as pediatricians in the future.

Thank you for your interest,
Ashaunta T. Anderson, MD, MPH, MSHS
Nina L. Shapiro, MD
Stephen C. Aronoff, MD, MBA
Jeremiah C. Davis, MD, MPH
Michael Levy, MD

ACKNOWLEDGMENTS

As with other books in this series, we sought to gain insights from study authors. We contacted as many study authors as we could, for them to have the opportunity to review our chapters and make any valuable suggestions to our work. We were able to communicate with 41 study authors. We are ultimately responsible for the content of the book, but greatly appreciate and acknowledge here the original study authors' time, effort, and comments regarding our summaries of their excellent studies.

We would like to thank:

- M. Douglas Baker, MD, first author: Outpatient management without antibiotics of fever in selected infants. *N Engl J Med.* 1993;329(20):1437–1441; and Unpredictability of serious bacterial illness in febrile infants from birth to 1 month of age. *Arch Pediatr Adolesc Med.* 1999;153:508–511.
- Marc N. Baskin, MD, first author: Outpatient treatment of febrile infants 28 to 89 days of age with intramuscular administration of ceftriaxone. *J Pediatr.* 1992;120:22–27.
- Nancy Bauman, MD, Dept. of Otolaryngology, Children's National Medical Center, first author: Propranolol vs prednisolone for symptomatic proliferating infantile hemangiomas: a randomized clinical trial. *JAMA Otolaryngol Head Neck Surg.* 2014;140(4):323–330.
- Allan Becker, MD, Department of Pediatrics, University of Manitoba, first author: Inhaled salbutamol (albuterol) vs injected epinephrine in the treatment of acute asthma in children. *J Pediatr.* 1983;102(3):465–469.
- Gerald S. Berenson, MD, Director, Tulane Center for Cardiovascular Health, Tulane University, senior author: The relation of overweight

to cardiovascular risk factors among children and adolescents: the Bogalusa heart study. *Pediatrics*. 1999;103(6):1175–1182.

- Carrie L. Byington, MD, first author: Serious bacterial infections in febrile infants 1 to 90 days old with and without viral infections. *Pediatrics*. 2004;113:1662–1666.
- Joseph Carcillo, MD, corresponding author: Early reversal of pediatric-neonatal septic shock by community physicians is associated with improved outcome. *Pediatrics*. 2003;112(4):793–799.
- Brian Casey, MD, chapter reviewer for: A proposal for a new method of evaluation of the newborn infant. *Curr Res Anesth Analg*. 1953;32(4):260–267.
- Robert W. Coombs, MD, PhD, Vice-Chair for Research, Department of Laboratory Medicine, University of Washington, participant in: Reduction of maternal-infant transmission of human immunodeficiency virus by zidovudine. *N Engl J Med*. 1994;331(118):1173–1180.
- Ron Dagan, MD, first author: Identification of infants unlikely to have serious bacterial infection although hospitalized for suspected sepsis. *J Pediatr*. 1985;107:855–860.
- Mark R. Elkins, MHSc, Clinical Associate Professor of Medicine, Central Clinical School, The University of Sydney, first author: A controlled trial of long-term inhaled hypertonic saline in patients with cystic fibrosis. *N Engl J Med*. 2006;345(3):229–240.
- Daniel Elliott, MD, MSCE, first author: Empiric antimicrobial therapy for pediatric skin and soft-tissue infections in the era of methicillin-resistant *Staphylococcus aureus*. *Pediatrics*. 2009;123(6):e959–966.
- Joseph T. Flynn, MD, MS, Chief, Division of Nephrology, Seattle Children's Hospital, reviewer for: Primary nephrotic syndrome in children. Identification of patients with minimal change disease from initial response to prednisone. *J Pediatr*. 1981;98(4):561–564. Dr. Flynn also graciously reviewed: Potter EV, et al. Clinical healing two to six years after poststreptococcal glomerulonephritis in Trinidad. *N Engl J Med*. 1978;298:767–772.
- James K. Friel, PhD, MSc, first author: A double-masked, randomized control trial of iron supplementation in early infancy in healthy term breast-fed infants. *J Pediatr*. 2003;143:582–586.
- William Furlong, MSc, McMaster University, first author: Health-related quality of life among children with acute lymphoblastic leukemia. *Pediatr Blood Cancer*. 2012;59(4):717–724.

- Marilyn H. Gaston, MD, first author: Prophylaxis with oral penicillin in children with sickle cell anemia. *N Engl J Med.* 1986;314:1593–1599.
- Francis Gigliotti, MD, Depts. of Pediatrics and Immunology, University of Rochester School of Medicine, senior author: A single-blinded clinical trial comparing polymyxin B-trimethoprim and moxifloxacin for treatment of acute conjunctivitis in children. *J Pediatr.* 2013;162(4):857–861.
- Nicole S. Glaser, MD, Professor of Pediatric Endocrinology, University of California at Davis, first author: Risk factors for cerebral edema in children with diabetic ketoacidosis. *N Engl J Med.* 2001;344(4):264–269.
- Fern Hauck, MD, Spencer P. Bass, MD, Twenty-First Century Professor of Family Medicine Professor of Public Health Sciences Director, International Family Medicine Clinic, first author: Sleep environment and the risk of sudden infant death syndrome in an urban population: the Chicago Infant Mortality Study. *Pediatrics.* 2003;111(5 Pt 2):1207–1214.
- Frederick W. Henderson, MD, Professor, Department of Pediatrics, University of North Carolina, first author: The etiologic and epidemiologic spectrum of bronchiolitis in pediatric practice. *J Pediatr.* 1979;95(2):183–190.
- Alejandro Hoberman, MD, first author: Treatment of acute otitis media in children under 2 years of age. *N Engl J Med.* 2011;364(2):105–115; and Oral versus initial intravenous therapy for urinary tract infections in young febrile children. *Pediatrics.* 1999;104(1 Pt 1):79–86.
- Jessica Kahn, MD, Division of Adolescent Medicine, Cincinnati Children's Hospital, first author: Vaccine-type human papillomavirus and evidence of herd protection after vaccine introduction. *Pediatrics.* 2012;130(2);e249–e256.
- Tohru Kobayashi, MD, Department of Pediatrics, Gumma University Graduate School of Medicine, first author: Efficacy of immunoglobulin plus prednisolone for prevention of coronary artery abnormalities in severe Kawasaki disease (RAISE Study): a randomised, open-label, blinded-endpoints trial. *Lancet.* 2013;379(9826):1613–1620.
- Mininder Kocher, MD, MPH, first author: Validation of a clinical prediction rule for the differentiation between septic arthritis and transient synovitis of the hip in children. *J Bone Joint Surg Am.* 2004;86-A(8):1629–1635.

- Nathan Kuppermann, MD, MPH, first author: Identification of children at very low risk of clinically-important brain injuries after head trauma: a prospective cohort study. *Lancet.* 2009;374:1160–1170.
- Jacques Lacroix, MD, Professor, Department of Pediatrics, Université de Montréal, first author: Transfusion strategies for patients in pediatric intensive care units. *N Engl J Med.* 2007;356(16):1609–1619.
- Kreesten Meldgaard Madsen, MD, first author of: A population-based study of measles, mumps, and rubella vaccination and autism. *N Engl J Med.* 2002;347(19):1477–1482.
- John March, MD, Professor of Psychiatry and Chief of Child and Adolescent Psychiatry, Duke University, first author: Fluoxetine, cognitive-behavioral therapy, and their combination for adolescents with depression: Treatment for Adolescents With Depression Study (TADS) randomized controlled trial. *JAMA.* 2004;292(7):807–820.
- Dennis Mayock, MD, Department of Pediatrics, Division of Neonatology, participant in: Null D, Bimle C, Weisman L, Johnson K, Steichen J, Singh S, et al. Palivizumab, a humanized respiratory syncytial virus monoclonal antibody, reduces hospitalization from respiratory syncytial virus infection in high-risk infants. *Pediatrics.* 1998;102(3):531–537.
- T. Allen Merritt, MD, MHA, first author: Prophylactic treatment of very premature infants with human surfactant. *N Engl J Med.* 1986;315(13):785–790.
- Michael Moritz, MD, chapter reviewer for: The maintenance need for water in parenteral fluid therapy. *Pediatrics.* 1957;19(5):823–832.
- Karin B. Nelson, MD, and Jonas H. Ellenberg, PhD, first and last authors: Predictors of epilepsy in children who have experienced febrile seizures. *N Engl J Med.* 1976;295:1029–1033.
- Paul O'Byrne, MD, co-author: Early intervention with budesonide in mild persistent asthma: a randomized, double-blind trial. *Lancet.* 2003;361:1071–1076.
- Jack Paradise, MD, first author: Effect of early or delayed insertion of tympanostomy tubes for persistent otitis media on developmental outcomes at the age of three years. *N Engl J Med.* 2001;344(16):1179–1187.
- Morton Printz, PhD, co-author: Pharmacologic closure of patent ductus arteriosus in the premature infant. *N Engl J Med.* 1976;295(10):526–529.
- Heikki Rantala, MD, Dept. of Pediatrics, University of Oulu, senior author: Antipyretic agents for preventing recurrences of febrile

seizures: randomized controlled trial. *Arch Pediatr Adolesc Med.*
2009;163(9):799–804.

- Shlomo Shinnar, MD, PhD, first author: The risk of seizure recurrence
  after a first unprovoked afebrile seizure in childhood: an extended
  follow-up. *Pediatrics.* 1996;98:216–225; and last author, Long-term
  mortality in childhood-onset epilepsy. *NEJM.* 2010;363:2522–2529.
- George H. Swingler, MBChB, PhD, first author: Randomised
  controlled trial of clinical outcome after chest radiograph in
  ambulatory acute lower-respiratory infection in children. *Lancet.*
  1998;351:404–408.
- Richard J. Whitley, MD, Distinguished Professor of Pediatrics,
  Professor of Microbiology, Medicine and Neurosurgery, University of
  Alabama, first author: Vidarabine therapy of neonatal herpes simplex
  infections. *Pediatrics.* 1980;66(4):495–501.
- Cathy Williams, FRCOphth, Dept. of Ophthalmology, Bristol
  Eye Hospital, first author: Screening for amblyopia in preschool
  children: results of a population-based, randomised controlled trial.
  ALSPAC Study Team. Avon Longitudinal Study of Pregnancy and
  Childhood. *Ophthalmic Epidemiol.* 2001;8(5):279–295.

We would also like to thank Rachel Mandelbaum, BA (UCLA School of
Medicine MD Candidate 2017) for her meticulous help in several of the chapter preparations.

Allergy/Immunology
and Rheumatology

1

Efficacy of Immunoglobulin Plus Prednisolone in Prevention of Coronary Artery Abnormalities in Kawasaki Disease

The RAISE Study

NINA SHAPIRO

Findings from our randomized study show that combination treatment with intravenous immunoglobulin plus prednisolone is better than that with intravenous immunoglobulin alone in prevention of coronary artery abnormalities, reducing the need for additional rescue treatment, and rapid resolution of fever and inflammatory markers in Japanese patients with severe Kawasaki disease.

—KOBAYASHI ET AL.[1]

Research Question: Does addition of prednisolone to conventional treatment with intravenous immunoglobulin (IVIG) and aspirin reduce the incidence of coronary artery abnormalities in patients with severe Kawasaki disease?

Funding: Japanese Ministry of Health, Labour, and Welfare.

Year Study Began: 2008

Year Study Published: 2012

Study Location: 74 hospitals in Japan.

Who Was Studied: Children with severe Kawasaki disease, who received a Kobayashi risk score[3] of 5 points or higher (see Boxes 1.1 and 1.2), indicating a high risk of nonresponse to immunoglobulin therapy and subsequent coronary artery involvement.

Box 1.1 JAPANESE GUIDELINES FOR DIAGNOSIS OF KAWASAKI DISEASE

Infants and children under the age of 5 should satisfy either 5 of the principal symptoms of Kawasaki disease or 4 of the principal symptoms plus coronary aneurysm or dilatation.[2]

Principal Symptoms:
1. Fever persisting ≥5 days
2. Fever for ≤4 days shortened by early intravenous immunoglobulin therapy
3. Bilateral conjunctival congestion
4. Changes of lips and oral cavity (reddening of lips, strawberry tongue, diffuse injection of oral and pharyngeal mucosa)
5. Polymorphous exanthema
6. Changes of peripheral extremities (initial stage: reddening of palms and soles, indurative edema; convalescent stage: membranous desquamation from fingertips)
7. Acute nonpurulent cervical lymphadenopathy

Box 1.2 KOBAYASHI RISK SCORES WERE CALCULATED USING THE FOLLOWING CRITERIA

- 2 points each for:
  - Serum sodium concentration ≤133 mmol/L
  - Illness of ≤4 days at diagnosis
  - Aspartate aminotransferase concentration of ≥100 U/L
  - % neutrophils ≥80%
- 1 point each for:
  - Platelet count ≤30Å~10^4/μL
  - C-reactive protein concentration of ≥100 mg/L
  - Age ≤12 months

Who Was Excluded: Children with a prior history of Kawasaki disease or coronary artery disease before study enrollment, those who were diagnosed with Kawasaki disease 9 or more days after onset of illness, those who were afebrile before study enrollment, those who received steroids or IVIG within 30 days or 180 days respectively, and those with coexisting severe medical disorders or suspected infectious disease were excluded from the study.

How Many Patients: 248

Study Overview: See Figure 1.1 for a summary of the study design.

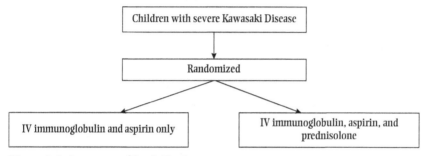

Figure 1.1 Summary of Study Design.

Study Intervention: Children diagnosed with severe Kawasaki disease were randomly assigned to receive either:

1. Conventional treatment with intravenous immunoglobulin (2 g/kg for 24 h) and aspirin (30 mg/kg per day until afebrile and then 3-5mg/day for at least 28 days after fever onset) or
2. The same regimen of intravenous immunoglobulin and aspirin just described plus prednisolone (2 mg/kg per day over 15 days) and famotidine (0.5 mg/kg per day), a histamine receptor antagonist, for gastric protection.

Follow-Up: Two-dimensional echocardiograms and laboratory data were obtained at baseline and at week 1 (6–8 days after study enrollment), week 2 (12–16 days after study enrollment), and week 4 (24–32 days after study enrollment).

Endpoints: The primary endpoint was the incidence of coronary artery abnormalities on two-dimensional echocardiography during the study period.

Secondary endpoints included coronary artery abnormalities at week 4 after study enrollment, need for additional rescue treatment, duration of fever after enrollment, serum concentrations of C-reactive protein at 1 and 2 weeks after enrollment, and serious adverse events.

RESULTS

The incidence of coronary artery abnormalities during the study period was significantly lower in the IVIG plus prednisolone group (3%) compared with the group receiving only IVIG (23%, $P < 0.0001$). At week 4 after study enrollment, patients in the IVIG plus prednisolone group also had significantly fewer coronary artery abnormalities, although the difference was less than that seen during the study period. Additionally, patients in the IVIG plus prednisolone group had more rapid fever resolution, lower incidence of rescue treatments, higher white blood cell counts and percentage neutrophils, lower aspartate aminotransferase concentration, higher serum sodium, higher total cholesterol, and lower concentrations of C-reactive protein.

Criticisms and Limitations: The RAISE study did not evaluate for many of the adverse effects of corticosteroids, though the study did identify an increase in the incidence of leukocytosis and high serum cholesterol in the group receiving prednisolone.

All study participants were of Japanese origin, and thus the results may not be generalizable to a more heterogeneous population. For example, the Kobayashi risk score was used to identify Japanese infants and children with severe Kawasaki disease that might be unresponsive to standard IVIG therapy, putting them at higher risk for coronary artery abnormalities. Yet, while this system predicted immunoglobulin nonresponse in Japanese patients, this scoring system has been found to have a low sensitivity for other populations, such as North Americans.[4] Further study is required to address the efficacy of the RAISE treatment regimen in non-Japanese patients with severe Kawasaki disease.[5]

Other Relevant Studies and Information:

- The Pediatric Heart Network (PHN) study, "Randomized Trial of Pulsed Corticosteroid Therapy for Primary Treatment of Kawasaki Disease," found no benefit of addition of pulsed high-dose intravenous methylprednisolone before conventional therapy with intravenous immunoglobulin with respect to coronary artery outcomes, reduction in adverse events, treatment time, or fever duration.[6]

This study evaluated the use of a single high-dose administration of corticosteroid in contrast to the RAISE study, which used low-dose corticosteroids over 15 days, but it highlights the controversy surrounding corticosteroid use in Kawasaki disease.

Summary and Implications: The RAISE study showed that the addition of prednisolone to standard of care treatment with IVIG and aspirin improved coronary artery outcomes, reduced the need for further treatment, and improved fever resolution in children with severe Kawasaki disease.

CLINICAL CASE: KAWASAKI DISEASE

Case History:
A 4-year-old male presented with a 5-day history of fevers to 103°F. Physical exam demonstrated an ill-appearing child with conjunctival erythema; dry, chapped lips; a swollen, red tongue; bilateral anterior cervical adenopathy; and a diffuse cutaneous exanthem. Laboratory testing was most notable for a sodium concentration of 130 mmol/L, C-reactive protein of 120, and a leukocytosis, with 85% neutrophils.

Based on this study, what would be the treatment of choice for this child?

Suggested Answer:
According to the RAISE study, children with a diagnosis of Kawasaki disease with a risk profile of >5 benefit from treatment including IVIG, aspirin, and prednisolone. This child's laboratory testing results included hyponatremia (2 risk profile points), elevated C-reactive protein (2 risk factor points), and neutrophil elevation (1 risk factor point), giving him a risk profile of 5, according to the RAISE study authors' criteria. This risk profile puts him at higher risk for coronary aneurysms. Addition of prednisolone to the IVIG/aspirin regimen in these high-risk patients gives them a significantly lower risk of developing coronary artery abnormalities, compared to children who received IVIG and aspirin alone.

References

1. Kobayashi T, Saji T, Otani T, et al. Efficacy of immunoglobulin plus prednisolone for prevention of coronary artery abnormalities in severe Kawasaki disease (RAISE study): a randomised, open-label, blinded-endpoints trial. *Lancet.* 2012;379(9826):1613–1620.

2. Ayusawa M, Sonobe T, Uemura S, et al. Revision of diagnostic guidelines for Kawasaki disease (the 5th revised edition). *Pediatr Int.* 2005;47(2):232–234.
3. Kobayashi T, Inoue Y, Takeuchi K, et al. Prediction of intravenous immuno-globulin unresponsiveness in patients with Kawasaki disease. *Circulation.* 2006; 113(22):2606–2612.
4. Sleeper LA, Minich LL, McCrindle BM, Li JS, Mason W, Colan SD, et al. Evaluation of Kawasaki disease risk-scoring systems for intravenous immunoglob-ulin resistance. *J Pediatr.* 2011;158(5):831–835.
5. Etoom Y, Banihani R, Finkelstein Y. Critical review of: Efficacy of immunoglob-ulin plus prednisolone for prevention of coronary artery abnormalities in severe Kawasaki disease (RAISE study): a randomized, open-label, blinded-endpoints trial. *J Popul Ther Clin Pharmacol.* 2013;20(2):e91–e94. Epub 2013 Apr 22.
6. Newburger JW, Sleeper LA, McCrindle BW, Minich LL, Gersony W, Vetter VL, Atz AM, Li JS, Takahashi M, Baker AL, Colan SD, Mitchell PD, Klein GL, Sundel RP; Pediatric Heart Network Investigators. Randomized trial of pulsed corticosteroid therapy for primary treatment of Kawasaki disease. *N Engl J Med.* 2007;356(7):663–675.

Behavioral

Measles, Mumps, and Rubella Vaccination and Autism

MICHAEL HOCHMAN, REVISED BY JEREMIAH DAVIS

This study provides strong evidence against the hypothesis that MMR vaccination causes autism.

—MADSEN ET AL.[1]

Research Question: Does the Measles, Mumps, and Rubella vaccine (MMR) cause autism?[1]

Funding: The Danish National Research Foundation, the Centers for Disease Control and Prevention, and the National Alliance for Autism Research.

Year Study Began: Data from 1991–1999 were included (the data were collected retrospectively).

Year Study Published: 2002

Study Location: Denmark.

Who Was Studied: All children born in Denmark between January 1991 and December 1998 (all Danish children are entered into a national registry at birth).

Who Was Excluded: Children with tuberous sclerosis, Angelman syndrome, fragile X syndrome, and congenital rubella—all of which are associated with autism. Children who emigrated or who died were also excluded.

How Many Patients: 537,303 children, 82% of whom received the MMR vaccine and 18% of whom did not.

Study Overview: The rates of autism among children who received the MMR vaccine were compared to the rates among those who did not (see Figure 2.1).

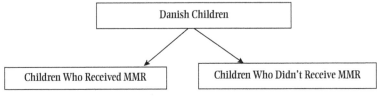

Figure 2.1 Summary of the Study's Design.

The authors used data from the Danish National Board of Health to determine which children received the MMR vaccine as well as the age of vaccine administration. The national vaccination program in Denmark recommends that children receive the MMR vaccine at 15 months of age followed by a booster at the age of 12 years.

Children were identified as having autism, as well as other autism-spectrum disorders, using data from a national psychiatric registry (in Denmark, all patients with suspected autism are referred to child psychiatrists, and when a diagnosis of autism is made it is entered into the registry). The authors also recorded the date when the diagnosis was made, allowing them to determine the time interval between vaccine administration and autism diagnosis.

Crude rates of autism were adjusted for age, sex, socioeconomic status, mother's education level, and the child's gestational age at birth.

Follow-Up: Children were monitored for autism from the time they reached one year of age until the end of the study period (December 31, 1999). The mean age of children at the end of the study period was approximately 5 years.

Endpoints: Rates of autism and rates of autism-spectrum disorders.

RESULTS

- Eighty-two percent of children in the study received the MMR vaccine, and the mean age of vaccination was 17 months.
- Among children diagnosed with autism, the mean age of diagnosis was 4 years, 3 months.
- The prevalence of autism among 8-year-olds in the study was 7.7 per 10,000 (0.08%), which was consistent with reported rates from other countries at the time.
- There was no clustering of autism diagnoses at any time interval after vaccination, nor was there an association between the age at which the vaccine was given and the subsequent development of autism. These findings do not support a link between vaccination and the development of autism (See Table 2.1).

Table 2.1. SUMMARY OF THE STUDY'S KEY FINDINGS

Outcomes	Adjusted Relative Risk of Autism Among Vaccinated vs. Unvaccinated Children[a] (95% Confidence Intervals)
Autism	0.92 (0.68–1.24)
Autism-Spectrum Disorders	0.83 (0.65–1.07)

[a]A relative risk <1.0 means a lower rate of autism among vaccinated children compared with unvaccinated children.

Criticisms and Limitations: The authors attempted to control for differences between vaccinated and unvaccinated children. Since this was not a randomized trial, the authors were unable to control for all potential confounders, which may have masked an increased rate of autism among vaccinated children. For example, parents of children with a family history of autism may have been more likely to withhold vaccination because of media reports warning about a link between the MMR vaccine and autism. As a result, children with a family history of autism—and presumably an increased risk—may have disproportionately opted not to be vaccinated, potentially obscuring an increased rate of autism due to the vaccine.

Although the authors did not identify a clustering of autism diagnoses at various time intervals following vaccination, the dataset did not contain the date when the first symptoms of autism were noted. Thus, it is possible that there was a clustering of first autism symptoms—but not diagnoses—at certain time intervals following vaccination.

Other Relevant Studies and Information:

- Children typically begin to show signs and symptoms of autism in the second and third years of life—shortly after most guidelines recommend that children receive the MMR vaccine. This may explain why some parents (and experts) link the vaccine with autism.
- Several other observational studies have also failed to show a link between the MMR vaccine and autism.[2-4] Several studies have also failed to show a link between thimerosal—a mercury-containing ingredient that used to be included in many childhood vaccines—and autism.[5-7]
- One widely cited article,[8] which was subsequently retracted by the journal that published it,[9] reported on a series of children who appeared to develop GI symptoms as well as signs of autism soon after receiving the MMR vaccine. The article generated considerable media attention as well as concern among parents; however the results have been widely called into question due to concerns about falsified data.
- Given increasing media concern regarding vaccine safety, the American Academy of Pediatrics undertook a systematic review of all evidence regarding vaccine safety[10]; their review also failed to identify any credible evidence linking MMR vaccination to autism.

Summary and Implications: This large cohort study did not identify a link between MMR vaccination and autism or autism-spectrum disorders. In addition, there was no clustering of autism diagnoses at any time interval after vaccination—which argues against a link between vaccination and the development of autism.

CLINICAL CASE: MEASLES, MUMPS, AND RUBELLA VACCINATION AND AUTISM

Case History:

Nervous parents bring their 15-month old baby girl to your office. Their previous pediatrician suggested that they find a new doctor after they declined MMR vaccination for their daughter. The girl's mother is concerned about the MMR vaccine because her sister developed symptoms of autism shortly after she was vaccinated. The parents want your perspective on the vaccine. Do you believe there's a link between MMR vaccination and autism? Will you care for their child if they decline vaccination?

Suggested Answer:

This study, as well as several others, have failed to show a link between MMR vaccination and autism. In addition, the most widely cited analysis suggesting a link between MMR vaccination and autism has recently been called into question due to concerns about falsified data. Although none of these studies has conclusively ruled out a very small link between MMR vaccination and autism, the preponderance of evidence suggests that there is not.

One way to respond to these parents would be to explain that numerous studies of high methodological quality have failed to demonstrate a link between the MMR vaccine and autism. While it is impossible to entirely exclude a very small association, it is very likely that there is not. You should also emphasize to the parents that there are clear and proven benefits of the vaccine, and that major professional organizations such as the American Academy of Pediatrics strongly recommend vaccination for all children. If the parents remain concerned, they might consider delaying vaccination for several months until the child is older.

If the parents opt not to have their daughter vaccinated, whether you will continue to care for their child is a matter of personal preference. Most physicians will care for unvaccinated children while continuing to encourage vaccination; however a small percentage choose not to.

References

1. Madsen et al. A population-based study of measles, mumps, and rubella vaccination and autism. *N Engl J Med.* 2002;347(19):1477–1482.
2. Taylor et al. Autism and measles, mumps, and rubella vaccine: no epidemiological evidence for a causal association. *Lancet.* 1999;353(9169):2026–2029.

3. Mrozek-Budzyn et al. Lack of association between measles-mumps-rubella vaccination and autism in children: a case-control study. *Pediatr Infect Dis J.* 2010;29(5):397–400.
4. Smeeth et al. MMR vaccination and pervasive developmental disorders: a case-control study. *Lancet.* 2004;364(9438):963–969.
5. Madsen et al. Thimerosal and the occurrence of autism: negative ecological evidence from Danish population-based data. *Pediatrics.* 2003;112(3 Pt 1):604–606.
6. Hviid et al. Association between thimerosal-containing vaccine and autism. *JAMA.* 2003;290(13):1763–1766.
7. Thompson et al. Early thimerosal exposure and neuropsychological outcomes at 7 to 10 years. *N Engl J Med.* 2007;357(13):1281–92.
8. Wakefield et al. Ileal-lymphoid-nodular hyperplasia, non-specific colitis, and pervasive developmental disorder in children. *Lancet.* 1998;351(9103):637–641.
9. Retraction—Ileal-lymphoid-nodular hyperplasia, non-specific colitis, and pervasive developmental disorder in children. *Lancet.* 2010;375(9713):445.
10. Maglione et al. Safety of vaccines used for routine immunization of US children: a systematic review. *Pediatrics.* 2014;134(2):325–337.

Treatment for Adolescents with Depression Study (TADS)

JEREMIAH DAVIS

... medical management of [major depressive disorder] with fluoxetine ... should be made widely available, not discouraged ... CBT should be readily available as part of a comprehensive treatment.

—THE TADS GROUP[1]

Research Question: What is the comparative effectiveness of cognitive behavioral therapy (CBT), a selective serotonin reuptake inhibitor (SSRI; fluoxetine), CBT and SSRI in combination, or a placebo alone in the treatment of major depressive disorder among adolescents?[1]

Funding: Contract RFP-NIH-NIMH 98-DS-0008 from the National Institute of Mental Health. Lilly, Inc. provided fluoxetine and matching placebo through an independent educational grant.

Year Study Began: 2000

Year Study Published: 2004

Study Location: Thirteen academic and community sites in the United States.

Who Was Studied: Volunteers between 12–17 years of age with a DSM-IV diagnosis of major depressive disorder, IQ ≥ 80, not currently taking any antidepressants, mood symptoms present in at least two of three locations (peers, school, home) for the prior 6 weeks before inclusion, and with a Children's Depression Rating Scale–Revised (CDRS–R) score of ≥ 45 (generally scores > 40 are consistent with depressive symptoms).

Who Was Excluded: Volunteers were excluded if they met any of the following conditions:

- Diagnoses past or present of severe conduct disorder, bipolar disorder, pervasive development disorder, thought disorder, or who were presently substance abusers or substance dependent
- Current use of psychotropic medications or receiving psychotherapy
- Failed two prior trials of SSRIs, or had intolerance to fluoxetine in the past
- Prior poor response to CBT as part of a clinical treatment program
- Pregnancy or refusal to use contraceptives, or other confounding medical condition
- Suicide attempt requiring medical care in the past 6 months, active ideation or intent, or suicidal ideation without a family able to monitor and guarantee adequate safety; they were also excluded if they had been hospitalized in the past 3 months for dangerousness
- Non-English speaking parents or patient

How Many Patients: 439

Study Overview: See Figure 3.1 for a summary of the study design.

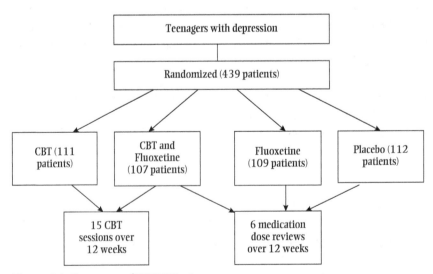

Figure 3.1 Summary of TADS Design.

Study Intervention: CBT: 15 sessions of 50–60 minutes over 12 weeks incorporating adolescent, parent and family, and combined sessions.

Fluoxetine: Six 20- to 30-minute visits with a single (consistent) pharmacotherapist distributed over 12 weeks. Starting doses of 10 mg/day were titrated if necessary to a maximum of 40 mg/day, based on Clinical Global Impressions (CGI) severity scores and the occurrence of adverse events.

CBT and fluoxetine: Both CBT and fluoxetine interventions; CBT modules and approaches were determined independently of any knowledge of medication changes.

Placebo: Same as fluoxetine alone group, but with placebo "doses" adjusted.

Follow-Up: Twelve weeks.

Endpoints: The authors assessed two major outcomes at baseline, 6 weeks, and 12 weeks:

1. Total score on the CDRS–R, which is a result of information gathered during parent and adolescent interviews
2. CGI improvement score measured at the end of treatment

Data were also collected from the Reynolds Adolescent Depression Scale (RADS) and the Suicidal Ideation Questionnaire-Junior High School Version (SIQ-Jr).

RESULTS

- Compared to placebo, fluoxetine with CBT ($P = 0.001$) had a statistically significant lower CDRS–R score at 12 weeks (33.79 for fluoxetine and CBT vs. 41.77 for placebo). Treatment with fluoxetine alone ($P = 0.10$) or CBT alone ($P = 0.40$) was not significantly different than placebo.
- Clinical responses defined by a CGI improvement score of 1 (very much improved) or 2 (much improved) are depicted in Table 3.1.
- Significance of these findings was estimated by calculating number needed to treat (NNT) for CGI improvement; for fluoxetine and CBT, NNT = 3 (95% CI, 2–4); for fluoxetine alone, NNT = 4 (95% CI, 3–8); and CBT alone, NNT = 12 (95% CI, 5–23).
- Suicidality (by RADS and SIQ-Jr scoring) decreased with treatment. Only the fluoxetine and CBT group was statistically significant in its

decrease compared to placebo ($P = 0.02$); fluoxetine alone ($P = 0.36$) and CBT alone ($P = 0.76$) were not.

- Regarding adverse events from treatment, a statistically significant elevated risk for harm-related adverse events was seen in patients receiving SSRIs (fluoxetine alone or fluoxetine with CBT), compared to those without SSRIs (placebo or CBT alone), with an OR = 2.19 (95% CI, 1.03, 4.62). Regarding suicide adverse events alone, too small a sample size (7 patients, 1.6% of total) attempted suicide to draw definitive comparisons; 4 of these were in the fluoxetine and CBT group, 2 in the fluoxetine alone group, and 1 in CBT alone. No patients committed suicide.
- Treatment with fluoxetine alone also showed a significantly elevated risk for all psychiatric adverse events (OR = 2.57, 95% CI, 1.11, 5.94); fluoxetine and CBT had an "intermediate" risk (OR = 1.45, 95% CI, 0.58–3.58).

Table 3.1 SUMMARY OF THE TRIAL'S KEY FINDINGS

	Clinical Response	
	Rate	95% CI
Fluoxetine with CBT	71.0%	(62%–80%)
Fluoxetine alone	60.6%	(51%–70%)
CBT alone	43.2%	(34%–52%)
Placebo	34.8%	(26%–44%)

Criticisms and Limitations: The study was composed solely of English-speaking patients, limiting application in other demographic populations. By excluding those with recent hospitalization, suicide attempt, or suicidal ideation without a safe family monitoring environment, the authors potentially biased their findings away from those at highest need for depression treatment, but these patients were deemed too unsafe to be randomized to a placebo group. The study intentionally did not include a "placebo and CBT" arm; placebo then became a trial-wide control. With the purpose of studying effectiveness (to guide clinical decision making), rather than efficacy (to allocate individual treatment effects), the design intentionally did not blind participants in the two CBT groups.[2] While the length of the study is relatively short, its participants were part of a later published longer time course spanning 36 weeks.

Other Relevant Studies and Information:

- The TADS group built on work done by Emslie et al.[3,4] on two separate randomized, placebo-controlled trials comparing fluoxetine to placebo alone in treating adolescent depression; prior to these studies tricyclic antidepressants had not been shown to be more effective than placebo, and behavioral/counseling strategies formed the basis of intervention.
- In a study with longer follow-up (36 weeks), the TADS group found that at week 36, rates of response on the CDRS–R were 86% for fluoxetine and CBT, 81% for fluoxetine alone, and 81% for CBT alone. Recipients of fluoxetine alone had less decrease in suicidal ideation than CBT or fluoxetine and CBT groups. Overall suicidal events were more common in those on fluoxetine alone (14.7%) than CBT alone (6.3%) or fluoxetine and CBT (8.4%).[5]
- The most recent guidelines suggested by the American Academy of Pediatrics recommend active support and monitoring for adolescents with mild depression; for those with moderate to severe, consultation with mental health professionals is recommended, and primary care clinicians should initiate CBT and/or SSRI medication.[6]

Summary and Implications: The TADS group found SSRI medication in combination with CBT in the treatment of adolescent depression to be effective and demonstrated a clear benefit of SSRIs above placebo. The study also highlighted the important side effect of more suicidal adverse events in those treated with SSRIs, and the protective effect of CBT on the occurrence of these adverse events. A longer follow-up study by the TADS group demonstrated combination therapy to be the most effective, but also revealed an equivalent level of response between CBT participants alone and SSRI alone at 36 weeks of treatment. These findings contributed heavily to the current approach for teenage depression which includes both medication and CBT focused counseling; data from this study also contributed to Food and Drug Administration warnings for all SSRI medications regarding increased suicidality in teenagers. This warning has become increasingly controversial after a decline in SSRI prescribing was followed by an increase in teenage suicide.

CLINICAL CASE: DEPRESSION IN A TEENAGER

Case History:
After a positive screening during a well child visit, your 14-year-old female patient admits to several months of depressed feelings and other symptoms; she has no psychiatric history and has otherwise been healthy. She admits to feeling hopeless and confesses that she has even thought about "ending it all"—though has no plan and has never attempted suicide. You make a diagnosis of major depressive disorder and she gives you permission to discuss your thoughts with her mother, who is very supportive; as a group you discuss management of depression.

Based on the results of the TADS group, should this patient be treated for major depressive disorder with medications, CBT, or both?

Suggested Answer:
The TADS group found that SSRIs (fluoxetine) in combination with CBT were the most effective treatment for adolescent depression, with over two-thirds of patients demonstrating a clinical response by 12 weeks of treatment. For this reason an SSRI and CBT are both recommended for moderate to severe depression in adolescents. Patients and families may prefer to start with one or the other treatment, but both modalities should be explained. In addition to discussing the most common side effects of SSRIs (headache, gastrointestinal effects, insomnia), it is also prudent to discuss the increased risk of suicidality in those taking SSRIs, relative to CBT alone. It's important in this situation to involve family members and caretakers who can assist the patient in monitoring for any increase in self-harm thoughts or concerns.

References

1. March J, Silva S, Petrycki S, et al. Fluoxetine, cognitive-behavioral therapy, and their combination for adolescents with depression: Treatment for Adolescents With Depression Study (TADS) randomized controlled trial. *JAMA.* 2004; 292(7):807–820.
2. March J, Silva S, Vitiello B; TADS Team. The Treatment for Adolescents with Depression Study (TADS): methods and message at 12 weeks. *J Am Acad Child Adolesc Psychiatry.* 2006;45(12):1393–1403.
3. Emslie GJ, Rush AJ, Weinberg WA, et al. A double-blind, randomized, placebo-controlled trial of fluoxetine in children and adolescents with depression. *Arch Gen Psychiatry.* 1997;54:1031–1037.

4. Emslie GJ, Heiligenstein JH, Wagner KD, et al. Fluoxetine for acute treatment of depression in children and adolescents: a placebo-controlled, randomized clinical trial. *J Am Acad Child Adolesc Psychiatry*. 2002;41:1205–1215.

5. The TADS Team. The treatment for adolescents with depression study (TADS). *Arch Gen Psychiatry* 2007;64(10):1132–1144.

6. Cheung AH, Zuckerbrot RA, Jensen PS, et al. Guidelines for Adolescent Depression in Primary Care (GLAD-PC): II. Treatment and ongoing management. *Pediatrics* 2007;120(5):e1313–e1326.

4

The Multimodal Treatment Study of Children with Attention Deficit/Hyperactivity Disorder (MTA)

MICHAEL HOCHMAN, REVISED BY MICHAEL LEVY

For ADHD symptoms, our carefully crafted medication management was superior to behavioral treatment and to routine community care.
—THE MTA COOPERATIVE GROUP[1]

Research Question: What is the most effective management strategy in children with attention-deficit/hyperactivity disorder (ADHD): (1) medication management, (2) behavioral treatment, (3) a combination of medication management and behavioral treatment, or (4) routine community care?[1]

Funding: The National Institute of Mental Health and the Department of Education.

Year Study Began: 1992

Year Study Published: 1999

Study Location: Eight clinical research sites in the United States and Canada.

Who Was Studied: Children between the ages of 7 and 9.9 years meeting DSM-IV criteria for ADHD Combined Type (the most common type of ADHD, in which children have symptoms of both hyperactivity and inattention). The diagnosis of ADHD was confirmed by study researchers based on parental reports and, for borderline cases, teacher reports. Children were recruited from mental health facilities, pediatricians, advertisements, and school notices.

Who Was Excluded: Children who could not fully participate in assessments and/or treatments.

How Many Patients: 579

Study Overview: See Figure 4.1 for a summary of the study design.

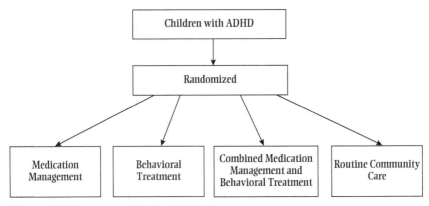

Figure 4.1 Summary of the Study's Design.

Study Intervention:

Arm 1: Medication Management—Children in this group first received 28 days of methylphenidate at various doses to determine the appropriate dose (based on parent and teacher ratings). Children who did not respond adequately were given alternative medications such as dextroamphetamine. Subsequently, children met monthly with a pharmacotherapist who adjusted the medications using a standardized protocol based on input from parents and teachers.

Arm 2: Behavioral Treatment—Parents and children in this group participated in "parent training, child-focused treatment, and a school-based
intervention." The parent training consisted of 27 group and 8 individual
sessions per family led by a doctoral-level psychotherapist. The sessions
initially occurred weekly, but were tapered over time. The child-focused
treatment consisted of an 8-week full-time summer program that pro-
moted the development of social skills and appropriate classroom behavior, and involved group activities. The school-based intervention involved
10–16 individual consultation sessions with each teacher conducted by
the same psychotherapist. Teachers were taught how to promote appropriate behavior in the classroom. In addition, children were assisted
daily by a classroom aide working under the psychologist's supervision
for 12 weeks.

Arm 3: Combined Treatment—Parents and children in this group received
both medication management and behavioral treatment. Information was
"regularly shared" between the counselors and the pharmacotherapists so
that medication changes and behavioral treatment interventions could be
coordinated.

Arm 4: Community Care—Children in this group were referred to community providers and treated according to routine standards.

Follow-Up: 14 months.

Endpoints: The authors assessed six major outcome domains:

1. ADHD symptoms based on parent and teacher ratings on a
standardized instrument called SNAP,[2] and
2. Five other outcome domains including:
   - Oppositional/aggressive symptoms based on parent and teacher
     SNAP ratings
   - Social skills based on parent and teacher ratings on the
     standardized Social Skills Rating System (SSRS)[3]
   - Internalizing symptoms (anxiety and depression) based on parent
     and teacher ratings on the SSRS as well as children's own ratings on
     the Multidimensional Anxiety Scale for Children[4]
   - Parent-child relations based on a parent-child relationship
     questionnaire
   - Academic achievement based on reading, math, and spelling scores
     on the Wechsler Individual Achievement Test.[5]

RESULTS

- At the end of the study period, 87% of children in the medication management and combined treatment groups were receiving medications, and of these children 84% were receiving methylphenidate while 12% were receiving dextroamphetamine.
- 49.8% of children receiving medications experienced mild side effects, 11.4% experienced moderate side effects, and 2.9% experienced severe side effects (based on parental report).
- 67.4% of children in the community care group received medications at some point during the study.
- ADHD symptoms improved considerably among children in all four arms during the study period; however, as noted below, children receiving medication management and combined treatment had the best outcomes.

Summary of MTA's Key Findings

MEDICATION MANAGEMENT VERSUS BEHAVIORAL TREATMENT

- Medication management was superior with respect to parent and teacher ratings of inattention and teacher ratings of hyperactivity/ impulsivity.

COMBINED TREATMENT VERSUS MEDICATION MANAGEMENT

- There were no significant differences for any of the primary outcome domains. In secondary analyses of global outcomes, however, combined treatment offered slight advantages over medication management alone, particularly among children with complex presentations of ADHD.
- Children in the combined treatment group also required lower average daily medication doses than those in the medication management group (31.2 mg vs. 37.7 mg).

COMBINED TREATMENT VERSUS BEHAVIORAL TREATMENT

- Combined treatment was superior with respect to parent and teacher ratings of inattention and parent ratings of hyperactivity/impulsivity, parent ratings of oppositional/aggressive symptoms, and reading scores.

COMMUNITY CARE VERSUS OTHER STUDY TREATMENTS

- Medication management and combined treatment were generally superior to community care for ADHD symptoms and for some of the other outcome domains.
- Behavioral treatment and community care were similar for ADHD symptoms; however, behavioral treatment was superior to community care for parent-child relations.

Criticisms and Limitations: While the MTA trial demonstrated the superiority of a particular medication management strategy versus a particular behavioral treatment strategy, medication management may not always be superior to behavioral treatment—that is, it is possible that a different behavioral treatment strategy might be equivalent or even superior to medication management.

The medication management and behavioral treatment strategies used in this trial were time-intensive and might not be practical in some real-world settings.

Other Relevant Studies and Information: After the MTA trial was completed, study children returned to their usual community care team for ongoing treatment. A 3-year follow-up analysis (22 months after the trial was concluded and children returned to usual community care) demonstrated the following:

- The percentage of children taking regular ADHD medications increased in the behavioral treatment group to 45%.
- The percentage of children taking regular ADHD medications decreased in the medication management and combined treatment groups to 71%.
- The percentage of children taking regular ADHD medications remained relatively constant in the community care group at 62%.
- Symptoms after 3 years were no different among the treatment groups for any measure—that is, the initial advantage of medication management and combined treatment was no longer apparent.
- Other studies have also demonstrated the benefits of stimulant medications in children with ADHD.[6–8]
- Guidelines from the American Academy of Pediatrics for children with ADHD recommend[9]:
  - medications and/or behavioral treatment for children <12 years depending on family preference
  - medications with or without behavioral therapy as first-line treatment for children 12–18 years (behavioral therapy can be used instead if the child and family do not want medications).

Summary and Implications: For children with ADHD, carefully controlled medication management was superior to behavioral treatment and to routine community care during the 14-month study period. This benefit did not persist 3 years after randomization (after children had returned to usual community care). Children receiving combined medication and behavioral treatment had similar outcomes as those receiving medications alone; however, these children required lower medication doses to control their symptoms. Despite its limitations, the MTA trial is frequently cited as evidence that carefully controlled medications are superior to behavioral treatment for children with ADHD. Nevertheless, behavioral therapy may be an appropriate and efficacious first-line therapy when the child and family prefer this approach.

CLINICAL CASE: MANAGEMENT OF ADHD

Case History:
A 6-year-old boy is diagnosed with ADHD based on reports from his teachers and parents that he has a short attention span and is hyperactive, sometimes disrupting classroom activities. His school performance has been adequate; however, both his teachers and parents believe he would perform better if his attention span improved.

Based on the results of the MTA trial, should this boy be treated for his ADHD with medications, behavioral therapy, or both?

Suggested Answer:
The MTA trial suggests that symptoms of ADHD are better controlled with medications than with behavioral therapy. Still, because medications may have adverse effects, the American Academy of Pediatrics recommends either medications, behavioral therapy, or both as first-line treatment for ADHD in children <12 years. Therefore, the boy in this vignette could initially be treated with either approach based on the preference of the family.

References

1. The MTA Cooperative Group. A 14-month randomized clinical trial of treatment strategies for attention-deficit/hyperactivity disorder. *Arch Gen Psychiatry.* 1999;56:1073–1086.
2. Swanson JM. *School-based assessments and interventions for ADD students.* Irvine, CA: KC Publications, 1992.

3. Gresham FM, Elliott SN. *Social Skills Rating System: Automated System for Scoring and Interpreting Standardized Test* [computer program]. Version 1. Circle Pines, MN: American Guidance Systems, 1989.

4. March JS et al. The Multidimensional Anxiety Scale for Children (MASC): factor structure, reliability, and validity. *J Am Acad Child Adolesc Psychiatry.* 1997; 36:554–565.

5. *Wechsler Individual Achievement Test: Manual.* San Antonio, TX: Psychological Corp, 1992.

6. Schachter HM et al. How efficacious and safe is short-acting methylphenidate for the treatment of attention-deficit disorder in children and adolescents? A meta-analysis. *CMAJ.* 2001;165(11):1475.

7. Biederman J et al. Efficacy and tolerability of lisdexamfetamine dimesylate (NRP-104) in children with attention-deficit/hyperactivity disorder: a phase III, multicenter, randomized, double-blind, forced-dose, parallel-group study. *Clin Ther.* 2007;29(3):450.

8. Wigal S et al. A double-blind, placebo-controlled trial of dexmethylphenidate hydrochloride and d,l-threo-methylphenidate hydrochloride in children with attention-deficit/hyperactivity disorder. *J Am Acad Child Adolesc Psychiatry.* 2004; 43(11):1406.

9. American Academy of Pediatrics. ADHD: Clinical practice guideline for the diagnosis, evaluation, and treatment of attention-deficit/hyperactivity disorder in children and adolescents. *Pediatrics.* 2011;128(5):1007.

SECTION 3

Cardiology

5

Pharmacologic Closure of a Patent Ductus Arteriosus in Premature Infants

MICHAEL LEVY

> *Dramatic clinical improvement was observed in each infant within 24 hours of indomethacin administration.*
>
> —FRIEDMAN ET. AL.[1]

Research Question: Does administration of the prostaglandin inhibitor indomethacin reduce or eliminate the clinical signs seen in patients with a symptomatic patent ductus arteriosus (PDA)?[1]

Funding: U.S. Public Health Service.

Year Published: 1976

Study Location: University of California, San Diego.

Who Was Studied: Premature infants with severe respiratory distress syndrome and prominent signs of left-to-right shunting.

Who Was Excluded: Patients with evidence of gastrointestinal bleeding, low platelets, abnormal coagulation studies, or hyperbilirubinemia >10 mg/dL.

How Many Patients: 6

Study Overview: A case series of 6 consecutive infants treated with indomethacin who otherwise would have had surgical PDA ligation.

Study Intervention: A single dose of indomethacin, either 5 mg/kg by rectum or 2.5 mg/kg by NG tube.

Follow-Up: Patients were followed up by physical exam and echocardiographic evaluation at 3, 6, 12, and 24 hours, and then daily.

Endpoints:

- Clinical signs of severe left-to-right shunting including bounding pulses, hyperactive precordium, cardiomegaly, and systolic murmur
- Progressive pulmonary edema on chest x-ray
- Left atrial/aortic root (LA/Ao) ratio, a marker of left-to-right shunting

RESULTS

- Five of 6 infants had complete resolution of clinical findings of PDA. The sixth had a persistent systolic heart murmur for 48 hours, but all other signs of PDA had resolved by 24 hours.
- The 4 infants on ventilatory support were extubated "without difficulty."
- LA/Ao ratios of each infant decreased significantly ($P < 0.001$) at 24 hours posttreatment.
- Two infants had statistically significant decrease in urine output along with increases in blood urea nitrogen and serum creatinine. Oliguria resolved in both patients within 72–96 hours and laboratory values returned to normal.

Criticisms and Limitations:

- As with all case series, there is risk of selection bias. The included patients may have been more likely to respond to treatment.
- The assessment of clinical improvement was based on subjective factors and introduces interobserver variability.
- There was no control group and so the patients may have had improvement without treatment.

- The patients were all ≥29 weeks gestation, and weighed >1,000 g. They therefore do not represent the more premature and smaller infants who are likely to be more ill and may have differing response to indomethacin.
- There is no consideration of the long-term benefit of PDA closure.

Additional Information:

- The effectiveness of indomethacin at closing the PDA in preterm infants was confirmed by a randomized trial comparing several treatment strategies that found that infants who received indomethacin had closure of a PDA twice as often as those who did not.[2]
- Persistent PDA is associated with, though does not necessarily cause, morbidities including more severe respiratory distress syndrome, prolonged assisted ventilation, chronic lung disease, necrotizing enterocolitis, and intraventricular hemorrhage.[3] Five trials have shown increased pulmonary morbidity among premature infants with at least 6 days of symptoms from a PDA. These infants required prolonged mechanical ventilation or supplemental oxygen, which could theoretically lead to an increased incidence of chronic lung disease.[4] A surgical study showed that infants weighing <1,000 g at birth had decreased risk of developing necrotizing enterocolitis with early PDA ligation.[5] In one retrospective study, adjusted mortality was 8 times higher in preterm infants with persistent PDA.[6]
- Conversely, a systematic review of 49 randomized controlled trials showed no reduction in mortality, chronic lung disease, or necrotizing enterocolitis in patients with closed PDAs.[7] Twenty-three studies failed to show a reduction in the duration of ventilator or oxygen support with ductal closure. While there has been decreased incidence of severe intraventricular hemorrhage with prophylactic indomethacin, this has not resulted in improved developmental outcomes.[8]
- Indomethacin has adverse effects including impairment of renal function, intestinal perforation, and platelet dysfunction, which may promote bleeding.

Summary and Implications: This study introduced the idea that pharmacologic closure of a PDA with prostaglandin inhibitors is possible, and described cases in which this treatment was associated with resolution of symptoms associated with a PDA. Prostaglandin inhibitors are still the mainstay of medical therapy for symptomatic PDA, although there is growing evidence that this treatment may not improve outcomes and treatment of PDA may not be necessary.

CLINICAL CASE: PREMATURE INFANT WITH A SYMPTOMATIC PDA

Case History:
You are caring for a newborn born at 27 weeks gestation in the neonatal ICU. On the second day of life the patient develops increasing ventilatory requirements, and has a systolic heart murmur and bounding pulses. An echocardiogram confirms a patent ductus arteriosus. How would you manage this patient?

Suggested Answer:
This patient has a symptomatic PDA and consideration should be given to intervening in order to close it. A persistent PDA is associated with increased mortality and morbidities such as chronic lung disease and necrotizing enterocolitis. Prostaglandin inhibitors are effective and could be considered as first-line therapy. However, prostaglandin inhibitors can have adverse effects, and there is evidence that closure of a PDA does not improve outcomes, so conservative management should also be considered. This may include fluid restriction, diuretics, and careful ventilator management.

References

1. Friedman WF, Hirschklau MJ, Printz MP, Pitlick PT, Kirkpatrick SE. Pharmacologic closure of patent ductus arteriosus in the premature infant. *N Engl J Med.* 1976;295(10):526–529.
2. Gersony WM, Peckham GJ, Ellison RC, Miettinen OS, Nadas AS. Effects of indomethacin in premature infants with patent ductus arteriosus: results of a national collaborative study. *J Pediatr.* 1983;102(6):895–906.
3. Benitz WE. Patent ductus arteriosus: to treat or not to treat? *Arch Dis Child Fetal Neonatal Ed.* 2012;97(2):F80–F82.
4. Clyman RI, Chorne N. Patent ductus arteriosus: evidence for and against treatment. *J Pediatr.* 2007;150(3):216–219.
5. Cassady G, Crouse DT, Kirklin JW, et al. A randomized, controlled trial of very early prophylactic ligation of the ductus arteriosus in babies who weighed 1000 g or less at birth. *N Engl J Med.* 1989;320(23):1511–1516.
6. Noori S, Mccoy M, Friedlich P, et al. Failure of ductus arteriosus closure is associated with increased mortality in preterm infants. *Pediatrics.* 2009;123(1):e138–e144.
7. Benitz WE. Treatment of persistent patent ductus arteriosus in preterm infants: time to accept the null hypothesis? *J Perinatol.* 2010;30(4):241–252.
8. Schmidt B, Davis P, Moddemann D, et al. Long-term effects of indomethacin prophylaxis in extremely-low-birth-weight infants. *N Engl J Med.* 2001;344(26):1966–1972.

6

The Relation of Overweight to Cardiovascular Risk Factors among Children and Adolescents

The Bogalusa Heart Study

JEREMIAH DAVIS

> ... *the use of overweight as a screening tool for risk-factor clustering may be particularly effective in the early identification of persons likely to develop [cardiovascular disease].*
>
> —FREEDMAN ET AL.[J]

Research Question: Can overweight status predict adverse risk factors (lipids, insulin, blood pressure) in children, and how sensitive is overweight categorization for detecting adverse risk factors?[1]

Funding: National Heart, Lung, and Blood Institute, National Institutes of Health grants HL 15103 and HL 3219, as well as funds from the Centers for Disease Control and Prevention and the Robert W. Woodruff Foundation.

Year Study Began: 1973

Year Study Published: 1999

Study Location: Bogalusa, Louisiana.

Who Was Studied: A community-based population of schoolchildren between 5–17 years of age were serially examined between 1973–1994; each examination captured over 80% of the total possible target population of children in Bogalusa. Anthropomorphic and laboratory data were collected in a majority of participants on at least two examinations. Determination of weight category was based on the final screening examination for each individual. A total of 9,167 children were included (4,789 boys and 4,378 girls).

Who Was Excluded: Subjects outside of the geographic catchment; those with nonfasting test values; or those without recorded values for height, weight, systolic blood pressure (SBP), and total cholesterol (TC).

How Many Subjects: 9,167

Study Overview: See Figure 6.1 for a summary of the study design.

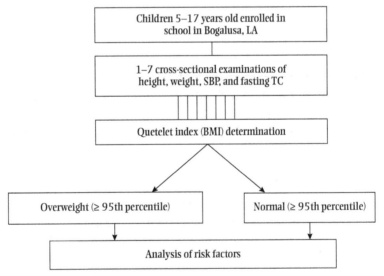

Figure 6.1 Summary of Study's Design.

Study Comparisons: Height, weight, and triceps and scapular skinfold thicknesses were measured at each visit. Risk factors for cardiovascular disease included: systolic (SBP) and diastolic blood pressure (DBP); fasting serum triglycerides (TGs); total serum cholesterol (TC); low-density lipoprotein cholesterol (LDL); high-density lipoprotein cholesterol (HDL); and serum insulin. Subjects were identified as overweight based on the Quetelet index (BMI) made at the last recorded examination for each participant. Subjects were classified as overweight if the BMI was ≥95th percentile compared to national benchmarks (Health Examination Survey II and III; National Health and Nutrition Examination Surveys I, II, and III). Since there is not an established abnormal level for serum insulin, a level ≥95th percentile adjusted for age, sex, and race was used as a cutoff.

Cardiovascular risk factors were dichotomized as "high" or "not high" using national standards (Table 6.1; HDL was dichotomized as low or not low).[2-4] It's important to note that these levels are no longer considered standard by today's guidelines. The prevalence rates for each risk factor were determined for the overweight (>95th percentile for BMI) and the non-overweight group (<85th percentile for BMI).

Table 6.1. DEFINITIONS OF ABNORMAL VALUES
AMONG RISK FACTORS STUDIED

Risk Factor	Referent
Total Cholesterol	>200 mg/dL
Triglycerides	≥130 mg/dL
LDL	>130 mg/dL
HDL	<35 mg/dL
Insulin	≥95th percentile[a]
SBP and DBP	≥95th percentile[b]

[a]Adjusted for age, sex, and race.
[b]Adapted from National High Blood Pressure Education Program.

RESULTS

- Eleven percent of the study population was found to be overweight (BMI > 95th percentile). When comparing those with BMI < 85th percentile to those with BMI > 95th percentile, overweight correlated to increased odds ratios (ORs) for every risk factor studied (Table 6.2).
- Those with a BMI below the 85th percentile had no difference in individual risk factors (total cholesterol, LDL, etc.); when the BMI > 85th percentile, prevalence rates of the examined risk factors increased, and rates were even higher for those with a BMI > 95th percentile.
- Sixty-one percent of overweight children between 5–10 years of age had 1 risk factor. When compared to children with lower BMI, those with BMI > 95th percentile between 5–10 years of age were more likely to have 1 (OR 3.8), 2 (OR 9.7) or 3 risk factors (OR 43.5).

- Fifty-eight percent of overweight children between 11–17 years of age had at least 1 risk factor. Compared to non-overweight children between 11–17 years of age, those with BMI > 95th percentile were more likely to have 1 (OR 2.8), 2 (OR 6.5), or 3 risk factors (OR 22.6).

Table 6.2. ESTIMATED ORs ASSOCIATED WITH OVERWEIGHT STATUS FOR ADVERSE CARDIOVASCULAR RISK FACTORS AMONG 5- TO 17-YEAR-OLD OVERWEIGHT CHILDREN (BMI > 95TH PERCENTILE)

Risk Factor	ORs (95% CI)	Sensitivity[a]
TC > 200 mg/dL	2.4 (2.0–3.0)	24%
TG > 130 mg/dL	7.1 (5.8–8.6)	47%
LDL > 130 mg/dL	3.0 (2.4–3.6)	28%
HDL < 35 mg/dL	3.4 (2.8–4.2)	25%
High levels of:		
Insulin	12.6 (10–16)	62%
SBP	4.5 (3.6–5.8)	34%
DBP	2.4 (1.8–3.0)	23%

[a]Proportion of subjects with the risk factor who were overweight.

Criticisms and Limitations: First, the study summarizes data from cross-sectional examinations and as such does not provide longitudinal information about participants, for example the development of new risk factors over time. Second, while the sample population represents >80% of the population of interest, a substantial portion of the population did not participate. Last, the breakpoints for risk factor values are based on adult populations.

Other Relevant Studies and Information:

- The same Bogalusa study cohort has been followed for years. Additional studies using this population have found earlier menarche in African American females,[5] increases in carotid artery intima-media thickness noted with elevated BMI and triceps skinfold thickness,[6] and most recently the relationship among various anthropomorphic measurements and risk factors for cardiovascular disease—ultimately reaffirming the use of BMI or waist circumference/height measurements.[7]
- Finally, studies from Bogalusa established associations among cardiovascular risk factors and atherosclerosis in childhood, linking childhood obesity and cardiovascular risk.[8]

Summary and Implications: This study and others demonstrate a strong association between childhood obesity and cardiovascular risk factors. It supports the utility of a simple office screen tool—calculation of the BMI—to detect clinically important risk factors for cardiovascular disease; while BMI is important, these studies also highlight the role of a multifactorial risk assessment including multiple pieces of data. The early recognition of overweight or obese status in children, and an emphasis on screening such individuals for aberrations in lipids and blood pressure in the hope of intervening early in life, may prevent morbidity in adulthood.

CLINICAL CASE: OBESITY AS A SCREEN FOR CARDIOVASCULAR RISK FACTORS

Case History:

An 8-year-old male presents to your outpatient clinic for a routine well child check. His BMI is calculated at the 97th percentile on a childhood curve. The remainder of his vital signs, including BP, are normal. The remainder of his physical exam and well child check are unremarkable and his immunizations are up to date. What recommendations should you make to his parents regarding his weight?

Suggested Answer:

In addition to addressing his obesity from a dietary and physical activity viewpoint, his elevated BMI warrants lab testing for dyslipidemia (even though guidelines don't recommend lipid screening for children of normal weight until age 9). Based on the findings of the Bogalusa cohort and related studies, it is clear that cardiovascular disease starts early in childhood and is linked with overweight and obese status. Obese young children should be monitored for early signs of comorbidities such as hypertension, insulin resistance, and hyperlipidemia.

References

1. Freedman DS, Dietz WH, Srinivasan SR, Berenson GS. The relation of overweight to cardiovascular risk factors among children and adolescents: the Bogalusa heart study. *Pediatrics.* 1999;103(6):1175–1182.
2. National Cholesterol Education Program. *Report of the Expert Panel on Blood Cholesterol Levels in Children and Adolescents.* National Institutes of Health publication no. 91-2732. Washington, DC: US Department of Health and Human Services; September 1991.

3. American Academy of Pediatrics, Committee on Nutrition. Cholesterol on child-hood. *Pediatrics.* 1998;101:141–147.

4. Kwiterovich PO Jr. Plasma lipid and lipoprotein levels in childhood. *Ann N Y Acad Sci.* 1991;623:90–107.

5. Freedman DS, Khan LK, Serdula MK, Dietz WH, Srinivasan SR, Berenson GS. Relation of age at menarche to race, time period, and anthropometric dimensions: the Bogalusa Heart Study. *Pediatrics.* 2002;110(4):e43.

6. Freedman DS, Dietz WH, Tang R, et al. The relation of obesity throughout life to carotid intima-media thickness in adulthood: the Bogalusa Heart Study. *Int J Obes Relat Metab Disord* 2004;28(1):159–166.

7. Freedman DS, Blanck HM, Dietz WH, DasMahapatra P, Srinivasan SR, Berenson GS. Is the body adiposity index (hip circumference/height(1.5)) more strongly related to skinfold thicknesses and risk factor levels than is BMI? The Bogalusa Heart Study. *Br J Nutr.* 2013;109(2):338–345.

8. Berenson GS, Srinivasan SR, Bao W, Newman WP III, Tracy RE, Wattigney WA. Association between multiple cardiovascular risk factors and atherosclerosis in children and young adults. The Bogalusa Heart Study. *N Engl J Med.* 1998; 338(23):1650–1656.

SECTION 4

Dermatology

7

Propranolol versus Prednisolone for Symptomatic Proliferating Infantile Hemangiomas

A Randomized Clinical Trial

NINA SHAPIRO

> *Based on similar efficacy between medications but the higher rate of severe adverse events with prednisolone therapy, propranolol should be considered the first line of therapy for symptomatic infantile hemangiomas if contraindications to its use do not exist.*
>
> —BAUMAN ET AL.[1]

Research Question: Is propranolol more effective and safer than prednisolone for treatment of symptomatic, proliferating infantile hemangiomas (IH)?

Funding: Eunice Kennedy Shriver National Institute of Child Health and Human Development of the National Institutes of Health and the National Center for Research Resources of the National Institutes of Health

Year Study Began: 2010

Year Study Published: 2014

Study Location: Children's National Medical Center, University of Iowa, and Johns Hopkins Hospital.

Who Was Studied: Infants aged 2 weeks to 6 months with symptomatic, actively proliferating IH. (Hemangiomas were considered symptomatic if they impaired function—e.g., leading to airway obstruction, dysphagia, visual disturbance, or hearing loss—were ulcerated, caused pain, or were in cosmetically sensitive regions.)

Who Was Excluded: Infants with nonproliferating IH or those who had received other treatment for IH were excluded from the study. Additionally, those with liver disease, abnormal blood glucose levels, hypotension, reactive airway disease, cardiac anomalies, and PHACE syndrome (*P*osterior fossa brain malformations, *H*emangiomas, *A*rterial abnormalities, *C*oarctation of the aorta and cardiac defects, and *E*ye abnormalities) with significantly narrowed intracranial vasculature were also excluded. Those with inadequate social support were also excluded.

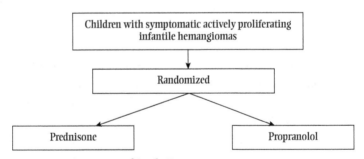

Figure 7.1 Summary of Study Design.

How Many Patients: 19

Study Overview: See Figure 7.1 for a summary of the study design.

Study Intervention: Children with symptomatic actively proliferating IH received either oral prednisolone (2.0 mg/kg per day) or propranolol (2.0 mg/ kg per day).

Follow-Up: 4 months

Endpoints: The primary endpoint was change in hemangioma size after 4 months of therapy with either prednisolone or propranolol. Blinded investigators measured total surface area, based on the outer margin of the hemangioma, and adjusted total surface area, accounting for central clearing within the margins of the hemangioma. Decline (involution) was defined as a reduction in size or percentage of skin involvement from the prior visit. Secondary endpoints included the rate of response to medication, frequency of adverse events, and severity of adverse events based on the Common Terminology Criteria for Adverse Events scale of 1 to 5 (1 = mild and 5 = fatal).

Results: Propranolol and prednisone were both effective in decreasing infantile hemangioma size. At 4 months, there was no significant difference between the treatment groups in proportional decrease of hemangioma total surface area and adjusted total surface area ($P = 0.12$ and 0.56, respectively). Patients in the prednisolone group exhibited faster decline in hemangioma total surface area compared with patients in the propranolol group ($P = 0.03$). However, when central clearing within the margins of the hemangioma was included in the analysis using the adjusted total surface area, no significant difference in response rate was seen ($P = 0.91$).

The frequency of adverse events was similar between the two groups ($P = 0.84$); however, the adverse events in patients taking prednisolone were more severe, principally associated with growth retardation (height and weight < fifth percentile) in 5 patients treated with prednisolone, and in 0 patients treated with propranolol ($P < 0.004$). These severe adverse effects prompted 75% of patients in the prednisolone treatment group to withdraw early from the study due to medication-related concerns. Patients taking propranolol had more pulmonary adverse effects, most of which were upper respiratory tract infections. Overall, adverse events in patients receiving propranolol were milder than those seen in the prednisolone group. No significant difference in the number of vascular adverse effects (reflected as blood pressure elevation or diminution) was observed between the two groups, and all vascular events were asymptomatic and resolved spontaneously. Based on the greater incidence of severe adverse effects associated with prednisolone, the Data Safety Monitoring Board terminated the study before targeted enrollment was reached.

Criticisms and Limitations:

- Even though this stu]dy provided evidence comparing the efficacy of propranolol versus prednisolone and the severity of adverse events from prednisolone, low study enrollment and early termination of the study prevented definitive comparison of prednisolone and propranolol for treatment of infantile hemangiomas. One explanation for low study enrollment is that one center lost its point of equipoise, and did not enroll any patients. The study investigators from that center felt that propranolol was superior to prednisolone soon after joining the study group; thus, they did not enroll any participants. As the authors stated, this information might be useful in the future should significant short- or long-term adverse effects from propranolol that might prevent its use be demonstrated.

- Due to the heterogeneity of hemangiomas, a long-standing issue in infantile hemangioma research was the lack of a validated, standardized, and reliable instrument to measure hemangioma severity. The Hemangioma Severity Scale and the Hemangioma Dynamic Complication Scale were developed by the Hemangioma Investigator Group Research Core, and these scales are a reliable tool for documenting the severity of infantile IH. The scale is based on size, location, risk for associated structural anomalies, complications, pain, and disfigurement.[2] At the time that the present study began, these tools were not available. The outcome of this study was based on total surface area and adjusted total surface area of the lesions, which may be unreliable for determining hemangioma severity and treatment response.

- While propranolol successfully reduced hemangioma size, the mechanism of action is unknown; the question remains whether propranolol only accelerates onset of involution or actually improves the final outcome of involution.

Other Relevant Studies and Information: There are currently no FDA-approved drugs for the treatment of infantile hemangiomas. Both prednisolone and propranolol are off-label therapies for this disorder.[3] Additionally, propranolol does not have an FDA-approved indication in pediatric patients and is not commonly used in children.[3] Therefore, there is a need for consensus protocols regarding dose, safety and toxicity, and use in patients with coexisting conditions. A consensus conference was held in Chicago in 2011 to issue recommendations regarding the use of propranolol for IH. A large-scale phase III clinical trial is needed to determine efficacy, optimal dosing regimens, and long-term safety.[3]

Summary and Implications: Prednisolone and propranolol showed no statistical difference in hemangioma surface area reduction at 4 months following treatment initiation. While prednisolone may result in a faster rate of involution, it is associated with more severe adverse effects, and therefore propranolol may be considered as a therapeutic option for the treatment of symptomatic infantile hemangiomas.[1,4]

CLINICAL CASE: INFANTILE HEMANGIOMA

Case History:

A 4-month-old healthy female with a progressively enlarging red, bulky, pigmented lesion of the right auricle presents to your clinic. She has no other skin lesions, and it appears to be most consistent with a hemangioma. The auricular landmarks have become indistinct, with hemangioma obscuring the entire auricle, and completely occluding the external auditory canal. There are some crusted areas of the lesion, with areas of skin breakdown, bleeding, and early ulceration.

What is your treatment recommendation?

Suggested Answer:

According to this article, the patient should be offered oral propranolol 2 mg/kg/day, divided in three daily doses. The family should be counseled that, although this agent is not FDA approved for this indication, it appears to be efficacious and safe. Cardiology clearance should be obtained and cardiac function should be monitored before and during therapy.

References

1. Bauman NM, McCarter RJ, Guzzetta PC, et al. Propranolol vs prednisolone for symptomatic proliferating infantile hemangiomas: a randomized clinical trial. *JAMA Otolaryngol Head Neck Surg.* 2014;140(4):323–330.
2. Haggstrom AN, Beaumont JL, Lai JS, et al. Measuring the severity of infantile hemangiomas: instrument development and reliability. *Arch Dermatol.* 2012; 148(2):197–202.
3. Drolet BA, Frommelt PC, Chamlin SL, et al. Initiation and use of propranolol for infantile hemangioma: report of a consensus conference. *Pediatrics.* 2013; 131(1):128–140. doi:10.1542/peds.2012–1691. Epub 2012 Dec 24. Review.
4. Léauté-Labrèze C, Dumas de la Roque E, Hubiche T, Boralevi F, Thambo JB, Taïeb A. Propranolol for severe hemangiomas of infancy. *N Engl J Med.* 2008 Jun 12;358(24):2649–51.

SECTION 5

Endocrinology

8

Risk Factors for Cerebral Edema in Children with Diabetic Ketoacidosis

JEREMIAH DAVIS

In this study, the children with diabetic ketoacidosis who had higher serum urea nitrogen concentrations and more severe hypocapnia at presentation than other children with diabetic ketoacidosis were at increased risk for cerebral edema.

—GLASER ET AL.[1]

Research Question: What demographic characteristics, biochemical variables, and therapeutics at presentation of diabetic ketoacidosis (DKA) correlate with the development of cerebral edema?[1]

Funding: Children's Miracle Network and Ambulatory Pediatrics Association.

Year Study Began: 1982

Year Study Published: 2001

Study Location: Nine tertiary care pediatric hospitals in the United States and one in Australia.

Who Was Studied: Children ≤18 years old who developed cerebral edema secondary to DKA at 10 pediatric centers between 1982 and 1997. Patients were retrospectively identified based on chart review showing DKA and cerebral edema, cerebral infarction, coma, seizures, or death, or who underwent CT or MRI imaging, intubation, or mannitol treatment. DKA was defined as serum glucose >300 mg/dL, venous pH <7.25, or serum bicarbonate <15 mmol/L, and presence of ketonuria. The diagnosis of cerebral edema was based on altered mental status and either one of two criteria: (1) radiographic or pathologic evidence of cerebral edema, or (2) improvement clinically after specific treatment for cerebral edema (hyperventilation or hyperosmolar therapy). Each case was compared with 6 controls without cerebral edema, also retrospectively identified: three "random" controls and three "matched" controls. Random controls were patients admitted for DKA randomly selected by a computer. Matched controls were admitted with DKA and matched according to age, onset of diabetes (new vs. established), venous pH, and serum glucose concentration.

Who Was Excluded: Children not meeting the definition of DKA, cerebral edema, or over the age of 18.

How Many Patients: 61 cases, 181 random controls, 174 matched controls

Study Overview: See Figure 8.1 for a summary of the study's design.

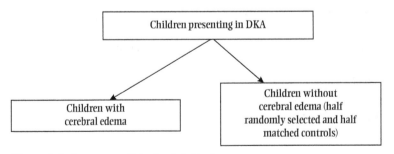

Figure 8.1 Summary of the Study's Design.

Determination of Patient Outcome: Records were reviewed for all children presenting with DKA at the study centers during the study period, including records from outside hospitals when referred to a study center. Similarly, all records of children who died at each center were reviewed to ensure no fatal cases of DKA-related cerebral edema were missed. Finally, all radiographic studies of children with cerebral infarction were evaluated by a neuropathologist and those found to be consistent with cerebral edema–related infarction were included in the cerebral edema cohort.

Correlation Methods: The authors conducted one-way analysis of variance for continuous variables and chi-square test for categorical variables between the cerebral edema group and both control groups. The random controls were compared to the cases using a logistic regression analysis of demographic and initial biochemical variables; the matched controls were compared using a conditional logistic regression analysis of demographics, biochemical variables, and therapeutics. Odds ratios were computed to estimate the relative risk. Finally, the multivariate analyses were tested to look for a statistically significant association in a majority of the iterations.

RESULTS

- Compared to the random controls, cerebral edema cases were younger, more likely white, and more likely to be newly diagnosed diabetics; additionally, these cases were more severely acidotic and hypocapnic, with higher serum glucose, serum urea nitrogen, and creatinine; compared to the matched controls, cerebral edema cases had higher serum urea nitrogen and lower partial pressures of arterial carbon dioxide ($PaCO_2$).
- Only serum urea nitrogen and $PaCO_2$ were associated with cerebral edema by multiple logistic regression analysis.
- In the conditional logistic regression analysis of cerebral edema cases versus matched controls, serum urea nitrogen, $PaCO_2$, rate of increase in serum sodium concentration during therapy, and treatment with bicarbonate were all significantly associated with cerebral edema (Table 8.1).

Table 8.1. Multivariate Analysis of Risk Factors for Cerebral Edema
in Cases as Compared to Matched Controls

Variable[a]	Relative Risk (95% CI)	P Value
Male sex	0.6 (0.3–1.4)	0.27
Age (per 1-yr increase)	0.9 (0.6–1.3)	0.53
Initial serum sodium concentration (per increase of 5.8 mmol/L)	0.7 (0.5–1.02)	0.06
Initial serum glucose concentration (per increase of 244 mg/dL)	1.4 (0.5–3.9)	0.58
Initial serum urea nitrogen concentration (per increase of 9 mg/dL)	1.8 (1.2–2.7)	0.008
Initial serum bicarbonate concentration (per increase of 3.6 mmol/L)	1.2 (0.5–2.6)	0.73
Initial $PaCO_2$ (per decrease of 7.8 mm Hg)	2.7 (1.4–5.1)	0.002
Rate of increase in serum sodium concentration during therapy (per increase of 5.8 mmol/L/hour)	0.6 (0.4–0.9)	0.01
Rate of decrease in serum glucose concentration during therapy (per decrease of 190mg/dL/hour)	0.8 (0.5–1.4)	0.41
Rate of increase in serum bicarbonate concentration during therapy (per increase of 3 mmol/L/hour)	0.8 (0.5–1.1)	0.15
Administration of insulin bolus	0.8 (0.3–2.2)	0.62
Treatment with bicarbonate	4.2 (1.5–12.1)	0.008
Rate of infusion of intravenous fluid (per increase of 5 ml/kg of body weight/hour)	1.1 (0.4–3.0)	0.91
Rate of infusion of sodium (per increase of 0.6 mmol/kg/hour)	1.2 (0.6–2.7)	0.59
Rate of infusion of insulin (per increase of 0.04 unit/kg/hour)	1.2 (0.8–1.8)	0.3

[a]For continuous variables (except age), increases or decreases are represented as 1 SD in the variable in the randomly selected control children.

Criticisms and Limitations: The definition of "cerebral edema" among the cases included altered mental status and one of two other criteria: (1) radiographic or pathologic confirmation, or (2) clinical improvement following specific therapy for cerebral edema (hyperventilation via controlled ventilation, hyperosmolar therapy). Given that some of the cerebral edema cases met clinical criteria alone and did not have radiographic or pathologic confirmation of actual edema, there is a possibility that some other process contributed to the altered neurologic status beyond DKA.

As is true for many pediatric studies, the population included is not large enough to detect significant associations of smaller magnitude, and therefore some of the variables listed as not significant may actually be significant, albeit with a smaller relative risk. Finally, little mention is given to pre-hospital care at outside clinics or institutions rendering other confounding factors uncontrolled.

Other Relevant Studies and Information:

- The authors utilized the same dataset to further examine risks for adverse outcomes among the 61 patients with cerebral edema and found that greater neurologic depression at the time of diagnosis of cerebral edema, elevated initial serum urea nitrogen concentration, and intubation with hyperventilation to a $PaCO_2$ < 22 mm Hg were all associated with poorer outcomes.[2]
- A similar study performed in Canada between 1999–2001 conducted prospective surveillance for cerebral edema associated with DKA, and then retrospectively assigned controls to identify risk factors. Examining 13 cases of DKA-related cerebral edema over the study period, the authors correlated lower initial bicarbonate value, higher initial serum urea concentration, and higher serum glucose concentration at presentation with DKA and cerebral edema; nonsignificant trends with higher fluid administration rates as well as bicarbonate treatment were found.[3]

Summary and Implications: Despite its rarity, cerebral edema in DKA is highly morbid and fatal when it does occur. For this reason, many studies have investigated which factors influence its development, and what criteria may be used to predict who will benefit from closer observation and specific therapy (i.e., in an intensive care setting). This study involved the largest retrospective cohort to date to objectively define variables associated with cerebral edema in DKA, and identified two key factors for cerebral edema in DKA: the initial serum urea nitrogen and $PaCO_2$. Additionally, administration of bicarbonate was found to convey a high risk for cerebral edema, and based on this study its use is now discouraged in children presenting with DKA.

CLINICAL CASE: CEREBRAL EDEMA
IN DIABETIC KETOACIDOSIS

Case History:

A community ED physician pages you overnight to discuss a 12-year-old male evaluated for abdominal pain, weight loss, and fatigue, and found to have a serum glucose concentration of 552 mg/dL with ketonuria. His initial arterial blood gas has a pH of 7.09 and a $PaCO_2$ of 17, and his exam demonstrates waxing and waning mental status, with periods of disorientation. In addition to initiating IV fluids and insulin the ED physician wants to know if you recommend a dose of bicarbonate to correct his acidosis.

Based on the results of this study, what recommendations do you make?

Suggested Answer:

Based on the findings by Glaser et al., this patient's initial $PaCO_2$ places him at increased risk for cerebral edema associated with new onset DKA. In addition to recommending against serum bicarbonate administration, it would be prudent to recommend transfer to a pediatric intensive care unit where serial neurologic examinations and neuroimaging can be performed and therapy specific for cerebral edema can be initiated .

References

1. Glaser et al. Risk factors for cerebral edema in children with diabetic ketoacidosis. *N Engl J Med.* 2001;344(4):264–269
2. Marcin JP et al. Factors associated with adverse outcomes in children with diabetic ketoacidosis-related cerebral edema. *J Pediatrics.* 2002;141:793–797
3. Lawrence SE et al. Population-based study of incidence and risk factors for cerebral edema in pediatric diabetic ketoacidosis. *J Pediatrics.* 2005;146:688–692.

SECTION 6

ENT

9

A Trial of Early Ear Tube Placement in Children with Persistent Otitis Media

MICHAEL HOCHMAN, REVISED BY NINA SHAPIRO

In children younger than three years of age who have persistent otitis media, prompt insertion of tympanostomy tubes does not measurably improve developmental outcomes.

—PARADISE ET AL.[1]

Research Question: Does early placement of ear tubes in young children with persistent otitis media lead to improved developmental outcomes (i.e., speech and language skills, cognition, and psychosocial development)?[1]

Funding: The National Institute for Child Health and Human Development, the Agency for Healthcare Research and Quality, and two pharmaceutical companies.

Year Study Began: 1991

Year Study Published: 2001

Study Location: Eight sites in the Pittsburgh area (2 hospital clinics and 6 private group practices).

Who Was Studied: Children between the ages of 2 months and 3 years who had a "substantial" middle ear effusion persisting for at least 90 days in the case

of bilateral effusion or 135 days in the case of unilateral effusion despite antibiotic therapy. In addition, children with intermittent effusion meeting certain
criteria (e.g., bilateral effusion lasting 67% of a 180-day period) were eligible.
Children were identified for the trial from a group of volunteer infants who
underwent regular (at least monthly) ear exams.

Who Was Excluded: Children with a low birth weight (<5 lb), those with a
major congenital abnormality, and those with other serious illnesses.

How Many Patients: 429

Study Overview: See Figure 9.1 for a summary of the study design.

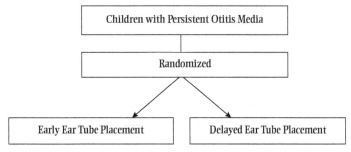

Figure 9.1 Summary of the Trial's Design.

Study Intervention: Children assigned to early ear tube placement were
scheduled for the procedure "as soon as practicable."
    Those assigned to delayed placement received the procedure only if a bilat-
eral effusion persisted for an additional 6 months or if a unilateral effusion persisted for an additional 9 months. Children in the delayed placement group also
received ear tubes at any point if their parents requested it.

Follow-Up: 3 years.

Endpoints: The authors evaluated the following developmental outcomes:

- Cognition, as assessed using the McCarthy Scales of Children's Abilities.[2]
- Receptive language, as assessed using the Peabody Picture
  Vocabulary Test.[3]
- Expressive language, as assessed by analyzing 15-minute samples
  of each child's spontaneous conversation (the authors recorded the
  number of different words, the mean length of utterances, and the
  percentage of consonants correct for each child).

- Parental stress, as assessed using parental responses to the Parenting Stress Index, Short Form.[4]
- Child behavior, as assessed using parental responses to the Child Behavior Checklist.[5]

In addition, the authors estimated the number of days that ear effusion persisted in the early placement versus delayed placement groups.

RESULTS

- The mean age at which children met the trial's entry criteria was 15 months.
- 82% of children in the early placement group received ear tubes by the age of 3 years, while 64% received ear tubes within 60 days of randomization.
- 34% of children in the delayed placement group received ear tubes by the age of 3 years, while 4% received ear tubes within 60 days of randomization.
- Patients in the early ear tube placement group had lower rates of persistent ear effusion than those in the delayed placement group; however, there were no differences in developmental outcomes between the groups (see Table 9.1).

Table 9.1. Summary of the Trial's Key Findings

Outcome	Early Placement Group	Delayed Placement Group	P Value
Percentage of children with ear effusion >50% of days during the first 12 months of trial	14%	45%	<0.001
Mean percentage of days with ear effusion			
during first 12 months	29%	48%	<0.001
during first 24 months	30%	40%	<0.001
Mean General Cognitive Index Score[a]	99	101	Nonsignificant[c]
Mean Receptive Language Score[a]	92	92	Nonsignificant[c]
Mean Number of Different Words[a]	124	126	Nonsignificant[c]
Mean Parental Stress Index[b]	66	68	Nonsignificant[c]
Mean Child Behavior Checklist Score[b]	50	49	Nonsignificant[c]

[a]Higher scores signify more favorable results.
[b]Lower scores signify more favorable results.
[c]P values not reported.

Criticisms and Limitations: Children in the delayed placement group had a higher rate of persistent ear effusion, which in most cases was accompanied by conductive hearing loss. Even though the hearing of children in the delayed placement group was temporarily impaired, this did not affect developmental outcomes.

Other Relevant Studies and Information:
- The authors continued to follow children in this trial for several additional years, monitoring developmental outcomes including auditory processing, literacy, attention, social skills, and academic achievement. During follow-up, no differences were noted between children in the early versus delayed tube placement groups at the ages of 4 years,[6] 6 years,[7] and 9–11 years.[8]
- A clinical practice guideline from the American Academies of Pediatrics, Family Physicians, and Otolaryngology-Head and Neck Surgery recommends that for persistent effusion in otherwise asymptomatic children 2 months to 12 years who are not at risk of speech, language, or learning problems and who do not have "considerable" hearing loss, intervention is unnecessary even if effusion persists for >3 months. Instead, the guideline recommends that such children be reexamined at 3- to 6-month intervals until effusion is no longer present.[9] Previous guidelines, issued prior to publication of this trial by the US Agency for Health Care Policy and Research, recommended ear tube placement for effusion lasting 4–6 months in all children 1–3 years with any degree of bilateral hearing loss.[10]
- Studies have suggested that ear tubes are frequently placed in children unnecessarily.[11]

Summary and Implications: Although children with otitis media and persistent ear effusion who received early ear tube placement had lower rates of persistent effusion than did children who received delayed or no tube placement, developmental outcomes were no different in the two groups. In addition, children in the delayed placement group underwent considerably fewer ear tube procedures.

CLINICAL CASE: EAR TUBE PLACEMENT IN CHILDREN WITH PERSISTENT OTITIS MEDIA

Case History:

A 2-year-old boy is brought to your office by his parents 3 months after he was treated for acute otitis media. He also was treated for acute otitis media at the age of 1 year. The boy is doing much better now, and has achieved all of his developmental milestones including language acquisition. On examination of his ears, you note that the tympanic membrane of the affected ear is no longer red or bulging; however, he has a bilateral effusion.

Based on the results of this trial, how should you treat his effusion?

Suggested Answer:

This trial found that early placement of ear tubes did not lead to improved developmental outcomes. Since the boy in this vignette is similar to the children included in this trial and is apparently asymptomatic, he should be observed for at least several additional months before considering ear tube placement. If the effusion persists for a longer period, or if he develops learning difficulties, substantial hearing loss, or repeated episodes of acute middle ear infection, ear tube placement should be considered.

References

1. Paradise JL et al. Effect of early or delayed insertion of tympanostomy tubes for persistent otitis media on developmental outcomes at the age of three years. *N Engl J Med.* 2001;344(16):1179–1187.

2. McCarthy D. *Manual for the McCarthy Scales of Children's Abilities.* San Antonio, TX: Psychological Corporation, 1972.

3. Dunn LM, Dunn LM. *Peabody Picture Vocabulary Test—Revised: manual for forms L and M.* Circle Pines, MN: American Guidance Service, 1981.

4. Abidin RR. *Parenting Stress Index: professional manual.* 3rd ed. Odessa, FL: Psychological Assessment Resources, 1995.

5. Achenbach TM. *Manual for the Child Behavior Checklist/2-3 and 1992 profile.* Burlington: University of Vermont Department of Psychiatry, 1992.

6. Paradise JL et al. Otitis media and tympanostomy tube insertion during the first three years of life: developmental outcomes at the age of four years. *Pediatrics.* 2003;112:265–277.

7. Paradise JL et al. Developmental outcomes after early or delayed insertion of tympanostomy tubes. *N Engl J Med.* 2005;353:576–586.

8. Paradise JL et al. Tympanostomy tubes and developmental outcomes at 9 to 11 years of age. *N Engl J Med.* 2007;356(3):248–261.

9. American Academy of Family Physicians; American Academy of Otolaryngology—Head and Neck Surgery; American Academy of Pediatrics Subcommittee on Otitis Media with Effusion. Otitis media with effusion. *Pediatrics.* 2004;113(5):1412–1429.

10. Stool S et al. *Otitis media with effusion in young children.* Clinical Practice Guideline, no. 12. Rockville, MD: Agency for Health Care Policy and Research, July 1994. (AHCPR publication no. 94-0622).

11. Keyhani S et al. Overuse of tympanostomy tubes in New York metropolitan area: evidence from five hospital cohort. *BMJ.* 2008;337:a1607. doi:10.1136/bmj.a1607.

General Pediatrics

10

Maintenance IV Fluid Requirements

MICHAEL LEVY

For weights ranging from 0 to 10 kg, the caloric expenditure is 100 cal/ kg/day; from 10 to 20 kg the caloric expenditure is 1000 cal plus 50 cal/ kg for each kilogram of body weight more than 10; over 20 kg the caloric expenditure is 1500 cal plus 20 cal/kg for each kilogram more than 20. . . . Maintenance requirements of sodium, chloride, and potassium are 3.0, 2.0, and 2.0 mEq/100 cal/day, respectively.

—HOLLIDAY AND SEGAR[1]

Research Question: What are the water and electrolyte requirements to meet physiologic losses?

Funding: Riley Memorial Association.

Year Published: 1957

Study Overview: This is not a clinical trial, but rather a classic practice guideline. The authors present a literature review and calculate a simplified set of recommendations.

RESULTS

This paper is the source of the ubiquitous "100-50-20 rule" for calculating maintenance IV fluid requirements; that is, 100 cc/kg/day for the first 10 kg body weight, 50 cc/kg/day for the next 10 kg, and 20 cc/kg/day for each subsequent kilogram. This rule produces a total daily fluid volume midway between the basal metabolic rate and estimated expenditure with normal activity previously published (see Figure 10.1).[2] There is also an adjustment for infants and smaller children, who are assumed to have near-normal activity while hospitalized and thus require maintenance fluid volume closer to that required with normal activity. The assumptions made in the generation of this rule are "necessarily arbitrary" as the authors concede.

The paper also presents suggested maintenance electrolyte needs. Given a paucity of data, the authors derive their recommendations by averaging prior suggestions from Darrow[3] and Welt.[4] As these averaged values fall between the electrolyte contents of human milk and cow's milk, they are taken to be acceptable.

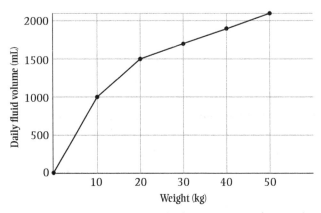

Figure 10.1 Maintenance IV Fluid Requirements by Weight.

Criticisms and Limitations: Holliday and Segar's 100-50-20 rule has been largely unchallenged for calculating daily total IV fluid volume for most pediatric patients, but there are patients for whom the calculation must be adjusted. The authors estimate that insensible losses constitute as much as half of the requirement. It follows that patients with increased insensible losses such as those with fever or burns may need more IV fluids, while those with decreased insensible losses such as patients on ventilators using humidified air or infants in humidity-controlled incubators may need less. Urinary water losses are estimated as half to two-thirds of maintenance requirement, so patients who are oliguric will need decreased maintenance rates.

Their published electrolyte requirements have recently come into question. Using their data, the maintenance IV fluid for a child will be hypotonic with respect to sodium concentration. In the example of a 30 kg child, the 100-50-20 rule gives us 1,750 mL per day, and at 3 mEq Na/kg/day or 90 mEq, the concentration of fluid would be 51 mEq Na per liter. Rounding this figure up to the nearest readily available solution suggests that ½ normal saline (77 mEq/L) should be the fluid of choice. An even more hypotonic fluid is called for in infants weighing <10 kg, where a similar calculation yields a solution of 30 mEq Na/L, or ¼ normal saline (34 mEq Na/L).

Beginning in the 1990s, hypotremia associated with hypotonic maintenance fluids was increasingly recognized and described. In February 2003, Moritz and Ayus[5] collected a series of >50 cases of neurologic morbidity and mortality in hospitalized children receiving hypotonic maintenance fluids. Many hospitalized children have conditions that lead to the syndrome of inappropriate antidiuretic hormone (SIADH). These include pulmonary and CNS conditions, pain, emesis, and stress. SIADH causes free water retention and natriuresis, and children are especially sensitive to the resulting hyponatremia. These authors argue that the excess free water of hypotonic fluids is not necessary in the absence of ongoing free water losses, and therefore recommended isotonic fluid for most hospitalized children receiving maintenance IV fluids.

This generated a controversy. Holliday and Segar[6] responded that initial volume expansion with normal saline will minimize the stimulus for ADH secretion, and they note the risk of hypernatremia from excess salt intake. Hatherill[7] argued that by increasing the sodium concentration of maintenance fluids, a total sodium deficit is implied. A more likely culprit is an excess free water load, prescribed because the 100-50-20 rule overestimates the water requirements of hospitalized children.

Other Relevant Studies and Information:

- Two recent meta-analyses[8,9] concluded that hypotonic maintenance fluids increase the risk of hyponatremia. The effect is seen most consistently in postsurgical patients and those in intensive care settings.
- It should be noted that no studies have demonstrated harm from isotonic maintenance fluids. However, this topic remains an active area of investigation.

Summary and Implications: The maintenance requirements for water can be readily calculated using the 100-50-20 rule, or 100 cc/kg/day for the first 10 kg body weight, 50 cc/kg/day for the next 10 kg, and 20 cc/kg/day for each kg thereafter. Sodium content of maintenance fluids can be estimated at 3 mEq/kg/day of sodium, 2 mEq/kg/day chloride, and 2 mEq/kg/day potassium, although the sodium concentration of maintenance IV fluids may need to be altered, and certainly warrants further study.

CLINICAL CASE: MAINTENANCE IV FLUIDS
FOR A HOSPITALIZED CHILD

Case History:
An 18-month-old girl is admitted to your general ward service with bronchiol-itis. She weighs 12 kg. She has been fluid resuscitated with boluses of normal saline in the emergency department and is now euvolemic. She is requiring supplemental oxygen via nasal cannula and is unable to tolerate oral intake due to respiratory distress and emesis. What IV fluids will you prescribe for her?

Suggested Answer:
Using Holliday and Segar's 100-50-20 rule, your patient will require 1,100 cc/day. If she requires 3 mEq/kg of sodium or 36 mEq total, then the sodium concentration of this fluid should be 36 mEq/1,100 mL or 33 mEq/L sodium. This corresponds with the readily available solution of ¼ normal saline (34 mEq/L). However, you remember that symptomatic hyponatremia has been associated with hypotonic maintenance fluids, and this patient has several potential causes of SIADH. Therefore you may also consider prescribing normal saline. This practice is supported by one recent paper demonstrating hyponatremia in patients with bronchiolitis receiving hypotonic fluids,[10] and another demonstrating worse outcomes for bronchiolitis patients with hypo-natremia compared to those with normal serum sodium.[11]

References

1. Holliday MA, Segar WE. The maintenance need for water in parenteral fluid ther-apy. *Pediatrics.* 1957;19(5):823–832.
2. Talbot, FB. Basal metabolism in children. In: *Brennemann's Practice of Pediatrics.* Hagerstown, MD: Prior, 1949, chap. 22.
3. Darrow DC, Pratt EL. Fluid therapy; relation to tissue composition and the expen-diture of water and electrolyte. *JAMA.* 1950;143(4):365–373.
4. Welt, LG. *Clinical Disorder of Hydration and Acid-base Equilibrium.* Boston, MA: Little, 1955.
5. Moritz ML, Ayus JC. Prevention of hospital-acquired hyponatremia: a case for using isotonic saline. *Pediatrics.* 2003;111(2):227–230.
6. Holliday MA, Segar WE, Friedman A. Reducing errors in fluid therapy manage-ment. *Pediatrics.* 2003;111(2):424–425.
7. Hatherill M. Rubbing salt in the wound. *Arch Dis Child.* 2004;89(5):414–418.
8. Wang J, Xu E, Xiao Y. Isotonic versus hypotonic maintenance IV fluids in hospital-ized children: a meta-analysis. *Pediatrics.* 2014;133(1):105–113.

9. Foster BA, Tom D, Hill V. Hypotonic versus isotonic fluids in hospitalized children: a systematic review and meta-analysis. *J Pediatr.* 2014;165(1):163–169.

10. Rodrigues RM, Schvartsman BG, Farhat SC, Schvartsman C. Hypotonic solution decreases serum sodium in infants with moderate bronchiolitis. *Acta Paediatr.* 2014;103(3):e111–e115.

11. Luu R, Dewitt PE, Reiter PD, Dobyns EL, Kaufman J. Hyponatremia in children with bronchiolitis admitted to the pediatric intensive care unit is associated with worse outcomes. *J Pediatr.* 2013;163(6):1652–1656.e1.

11

Predischarge Serum Bilirubin to Predict Significant Hyperbilirubinemia in Newborns

MICHAEL LEVY

> *...we have demonstrated the predictive usefulness and clinical value of universal bilirubin sampling in all term and near-term newborns...*
> —BHUTANI ET AL.[1]

Research Question: Can a predischarge serum bilirubin level predict subsequent significant hyperbilirubinemia in healthy newborns?[1]

Funding: Newborn Pediatrics Research Fund at Pennsylvania Hospital.

Year Study Began: 1993

Year Published: 1999

Study Location: Pennsylvania Hospital in Philadelphia.

Who Was Studied: Term and near-term newborns.

Who Was Excluded: Babies admitted to the NICU, babies with a positive direct Coombs test, and those requiring phototherapy before age 60 hours. Bilirubin levels obtained after starting phototherapy were not included in the nomogram.

How Many Patients: 2,840

Study Overview: Total serum bilirubin concentration was measured in newborns before discharge and again 24–48 hours after discharge through a hospital-supervised follow-up program. All values were plotted on an hour-specific nomogram and divided into the 95th, 75th, and 40th percentiles.

Follow-Up: 10 days

Endpoint: Significant hyperbilirubinemia, defined as greater than the 95th percentile.

RESULTS

- A nomogram (Figure 11.1) was developed, which tracked several percentile lines for hour-specific bilirubin concentrations.
- Predischarge bilirubin concentrations were then stratified according to this nomogram, and used to predict the likelihood of a patient subsequently developing a total bilirubin concentration >95th percentile (Table 11.1).

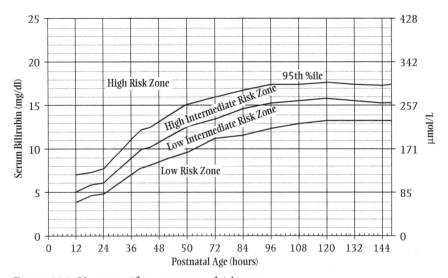

Figure 11.1 Hour-specific nomogram of risk zones.

- Phototherapy was initiated on 117 (4.1%) of infants. None of these infants were in the low risk zone before discharge. Of note, this study was conducted before the publication of the clinical practice guideline that suggested hour-specific treatment levels.[2] It is likely that many infants in this study treated with phototherapy would not require treatment according to current guidelines.
- No babies in the study developed total bilirubin concentration >25 mg/dL, required exchange transfusion, or developed signs of acute bilirubin encephalopathy.

Table 11.1. PREDICTIVE ABILITY OF PREDISCHARGE BILIRUBIN

Initial Risk Zone	Subsequent Significant Hyperbilirubinemia	Likelihood Ratio of Bilirubin Level >95th Percentile
High risk	39.5%	14.08
High Intermediate risk	12.9%	3.2
Low intermediate risk	2.2%	0.48
Low risk	0%	0

Criticisms and Limitations:

- Significant hyperbilirubinemia was arbitrarily defined as >95th percentile and is not necessarily predictive of clinically significant outcomes such as need for exchange transfusion or development of neurotoxicity.
- Only patients who complied with all requirements of the hospital-sponsored follow-up were included. Those who did not follow up may have been at increased risk for hyperbilirubinemia.
- The data may underestimate the probability of developing hyperbilirubinemia since patients requiring early phototherapy were excluded, though this accounts for only 18 newborns or <1% of the study population.
- 49% of study patients were exclusively breastfed. The rates of exclusive breastfeeding are higher now in most US populations[3] and exclusively breastfed infants are at greater risk for hyperbilirubinemia.

Other Relevant Studies and Information:

- One study of more than 300,000 infants found a 62% decreased incidence of bilirubin concentrations above recommended exchange transfusion levels for infants born in a hospital with universal predischarge screening.[4] Another study of more than 1 million patients showed that universal screening significantly decreased the incidence of bilirubin concentrations of 25.0–29.9 mg/dL, and of bilirubin concentrations ≥30 mg/dL.[5]

- Transcutaneous bilirubin measurements are as effective as serum measurements for screening, and this approach reduces laboratory costs.[6]
- Using total bilirubin concentration is an imperfect estimate of the risk of bilirubin neurotoxicity. Encephalopathy is not an outcome of published studies due to its rarity,[7] and not all children with bilirubin encephalopathy have a history of hyperbilirubinemia.[8]
- Some studies have shown universal screening increases costs[9] and utilization of resources such as phototherapy,[4,5] but these findings may be explained by preexisting trends in health care spending.[10] Universal screening does not appear to increase length of stay or subsequent hospital use.[10]

Summary and Implications: A predischarge bilirubin level can help predict a newborn's risk of developing significant hyperbilirubinemia. When used as a universal screening tool, fewer infants will develop high bilirubin concentrations. This benefit may be balanced by increased health care costs and an uncertain impact on the major outcome of interest, bilirubin encephalopathy. While not included in the AAP Practice Guidelines, a more recent report has recommended universal predischarge bilirubin screening for all neonates.[11]

CLINICAL CASE: PREDISCHARGE SERUM BILIRUBIN

Case History:
You are preparing to discharge a healthy full-term newborn from the nursery on the second day of life. A serum bilirubin obtained at 24 hours is 7.0 mg/dL. The baby has no risk factors for neurotoxicity. How likely is this baby to develop severe hyperbilirubinemia, and how should she be followed up?

Suggested Answer:
A bilirubin of 7.0 mg/dL at 24 hours of life falls into the high-intermediate risk zone on the nomogram developed by this study. Infants whose predischarge bilirubin is in this risk zone have a 12.9% chance of eventually developing severe hyperbilirubinemia. This risk is great enough to warrant repeating a bilirubin level, likely within 48 hours of hospital discharge.

References

1. Bhutani VK, Johnson L, Sivieri EM. Predictive ability of a predischarge hour-specific serum bilirubin for subsequent significant hyperbilirubinemia in healthy term and near-term newborns. *Pediatrics.* 1999;103(1):6–14.
2. Management of hyperbilirubinemia in the newborn infant 35 or more weeks of gestation. *Pediatrics.* 2004;114(1):297–316.
3. CDC Breastfeeding Report Card 2014. http://www.cdc.gov/breastfeeding/pdf/2014breastfeedingreportcard.pdf. Accessed February 12, 2015.
4. Kuzniewicz MW, Escobar GJ, Newman TB. Impact of universal bilirubin screening on severe hyperbilirubinemia and phototherapy use. *Pediatrics.* 2009;124(4):1031–1039.
5. Mah MP, Clark SL, Akhigbe E, et al. Reduction of severe hyperbilirubinemia after institution of predischarge bilirubin screening. *Pediatrics.* 2010;125(5):e1143–e1148.
6. Bhutani VK, Gourley GR, Adler S, Kreamer B, Dalin C, Johnson LH. Noninvasive measurement of total serum bilirubin in a multiracial predischarge newborn population to assess the risk of severe hyperbilirubinemia. *Pediatrics.* 2000;106(2):E17.
7. Trikalinos TA, Chung M, Lau J, Ip S. Systematic review of screening for bilirubin encephalopathy in neonates. *Pediatrics.* 2009;124(4):1162–1171.
8. Screening of infants for hyperbilirubinemia to prevent chronic bilirubin encephalopathy: US Preventive Services Task Force recommendation statement. *Pediatrics.* 2009;124(4):1172–1177.
9. Suresh GK, Clark RE. Cost-effectiveness of strategies that are intended to prevent kernicterus in newborn infants. *Pediatrics.* 2004;114(4):917–924.
10. Darling EK, Ramsay T, Sprague AE, Walker MC, Guttmann A. Universal bilirubin screening and health care utilization. *Pediatrics.* 2014;134(4):e1017–1024.
11. Maisels MJ, Bhutani VK, Bogen D, Newman TB, Stark AR, Watchko JF. Hyperbilirubinemia in the newborn infant ≥35 weeks' gestation: an update with clarifications. *Pediatrics.* 2009;124(4):1193–1198.

12

Sudden Infant Death Syndrome Risk Factors: The Chicago Infant Mortality Study

MICHAEL LEVY

Risk factors . . . demonstrated in this study must be addressed to reach the national goal of eliminating the racial disparity in [Sudden Infant Death Syndrome].

—HAUCK ET AL.[1]

Research Question: What risk factors contribute to sudden infant death syndrome (SIDS) in a minority population?[1]

Funding: The National Institute of Child Health and Human Development, the National Institute on Deafness and Other Communication Disorders, the Centers for Disease Control and Prevention, and the Association of Teachers of Preventive Medicine.

Year Study Began: 1993

Year Published: 2003

Study Location: Chicago, Illinois.

Who Was Studied: All infants who died from SIDS in Chicago between November 1993 and April 1996, and matched control infants. SIDS was defined

as "the sudden death of an infant under 1 year of age, which remains unexplained
after a thorough case investigation, including performance of a complete autopsy,
examination of the death scene, and review of the clinical history." The study
population was 75% black, 13.1% Hispanic white, and 11.9% non-Hispanic white.

Who Was Excluded: No cases were excluded.

How Many Patients: 260 cases and 260 matched controls.

Study Overview: The Chicago Infant Mortality Study conducted an in-depth
investigation into all SIDS cases of Chicago residents during the study period.
The study consisted of a scene investigation, autopsy, and interviews with the
family about medical history; sleep habits; tobacco, alcohol, and drug use; and
other factors.

RESULTS

- Case mothers were significantly younger, had less education, had less
  prenatal care, and were more likely to be single.
- The combination of prone position and soft sleeping surface was
  particularly dangerous, with an adjusted odds ratio of 21.0.
- Cases and controls both had higher rates of prone sleep positioning
  (57.3% and 35.0%, respectively) compared to the general population
  (25% in 2010[2]) (see Table 12.1).

Table 12.1. SUMMARY OF THE STUDY'S KEY FINDINGS

Variable	% of SIDS Cases	% of Controls	Adjusted Odds Ratio (95% Confidence Interval)*
Prone sleep position	57.3	35.0	2.3 (1.5–3.5)
Soft sleep surface	48.8	19.2	5.1 (2.9–9.2)
Shared bed	50.4	30.4	2.0 (1.2–3.3)
Ever breastfed	21.2	50.0	0.4 (0.2–0.7)
Pacifier use	15.0	31.9	0.3 (0.2–0.5)

*Adjusted odds ratios controlled for maternal age, education, prenatal care, and
marital status.

Criticisms and Limitations:

- Recall bias could affect the results if mothers of SIDS cases reported
  risk factors differently than mothers of controls.

- Additional risk factors would not have been found if they were not discussed in the interviews.
- The findings in this population may not be generalizable to different demographics or regions.

Additional Information:

- The findings in this study are consistent with AAP guidelines, which recommend supine sleep, firm sleep surface, room sharing without bed sharing, breastfeeding, regular prenatal care, and consideration of pacifier use. Other recommendations include removing soft objects and loose bedding from the crib, avoiding smoke exposure, and avoiding overheating.[3]
- The results of the Chicago Infant Mortality Study led to a multifaceted educational intervention targeted at the city's black population, and in subsequent years the SIDS rate declined more rapidly among that group than the general population.

Summary and Implications: This study was one of the largest and most comprehensive examinations of the sleep environment and risk for SIDS in a minority population. It was among the first to confirm the association between prone sleep position and SIDS in a US population. It was the first to suggest the additive effect of prone positioning and soft sleep surface.

CLINICAL CASE: SIDS RISK FACTORS

Case History:
You are working in a practice that sees a mostly black population. When counseling parents of newborns, you spend a considerable amount of time discussing SIDS prevention as you know that your patients are more likely to die of SIDS than the general population. What risk factors may be more likely in your patients that you could focus on in your discussion?

Suggested Answer:
This large study of a primarily black population showed significant risk from prone sleep positioning, soft sleep surface, and bed sharing. These may be high-yield areas of focus. Based on the results of this study, you would also want to encourage breastfeeding, and point out that pacifier use may be protective—though introduction of the pacifier should be delayed until breastfeeding is fully established.[3,4]

References

1. Hauck FR, Herman SM, Donovan M, et al. Sleep environment and the risk of sudden infant death syndrome in an urban population: the Chicago Infant Mortality Study. *Pediatrics*. 2003;111(5 Pt 2):1207–1214.
2. Moon RY. SIDS and other sleep-related infant deaths: expansion of recommendations for a safe infant sleeping environment. *Pediatrics*. 2011;128(5): e1341–e1367.
3. Moon RY. SIDS and other sleep-related infant deaths: expansion of recommendations for a safe infant sleeping environment. *Pediatrics*. 2011;128(5):1030–1039.
4. Howard CR, Howard FM, Lanphear B, et al. Randomized clinical trial of pacifier use and bottle-feeding or cupfeeding and their effect on breastfeeding. *Pediatrics*. 2003;111(3):511–518.

13

Treatment of Acute Otitis Media in Children

MICHAEL HOCHMAN, REVISED BY NINA SHAPIRO

[A]mong children 6 to 23 months of age with acute otitis media, treatment with amoxicillin-clavulanate for 10 days affords a measurable short-term benefit . . . The benefit must be weighed against concern not only about the side effects of the medication but also about the . . . emergence of bacterial resistance. These considerations underscore the need to restrict treatment to children whose illness is diagnosed with the use of stringent criteria.

—HOBERMAN ET AL.[1]

Research Question: Should children under 2 years of age with acute otitis media be treated immediately with antibiotics?[1]

Funding: The National Institute of Allergy and Infectious Diseases.

Year Study Began: 2006

Year Study Published: 2011

Study Location: The Children's Hospital of Pittsburgh and Armstrong Pediatrics (a private practice in Pennsylvania).

Who Was Studied: Children 6–23 months of age with acute otitis media. To qualify, children were required to have:

- Onset of acute otitis media symptoms within the previous 48 hours
- A score of ≥3 on the Acute Otitis Media Severity of Symptoms scale (AOM-SOS), which is scored from 0–14 based on parental reports of: "tugging of ears, crying, irritability, difficulty sleeping, diminished activity, diminished appetite, and fever"
- Middle-ear effusion
- Moderate or severe "bulging of the tympanic membrane or slight bulging accompanied by either otalgia or marked erythema of the membrane"

Who Was Excluded: Children with another illness such as pneumonia or cystic fibrosis, those who had not yet received at least two doses of the pneumococcal conjugate vaccine, those with an allergy to amoxicillin, those with recent antibiotic exposure, and those with a ruptured tympanic membrane.

How Many Patients: 291

Study Overview: See Figure 13.1 for a summary of the trial's design.

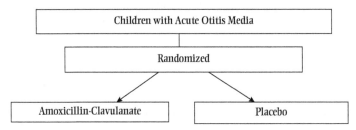

Figure 13.1 Summary of the Trial's Design.

Study Intervention: Children assigned to the antibiotic group received amoxicillin-clavulanate in 2 divided doses for 10 days (total daily dose 90 mg/kg of amoxicillin and 6.4 mg/kg of clavulanate). Children assigned to the control group received a placebo suspension twice daily for 10 days.

Follow-Up: Evaluations were conducted at various time intervals during the first 21–25 days after enrollment.

Endpoints: Primary outcomes: Time to symptom resolution and symptom burden. Secondary outcomes: clinical failure, adverse events, and health care resource utilization.

RESULTS

- At baseline, the mean AOM-SOS score was 7.8, and 52% of children had bilateral disease; in addition, 72% of children had moderate or severe bulging of the tympanic membrane.
- Sustained symptom resolution occurred more quickly in the antibiotic group and symptom burden was lower in the antibiotic group; however, there were more antibiotic-related complications in the antibiotic group (see Table 13.1).
- Treatment with amoxicillin-clavulanate resulted in the greatest absolute benefit among children with the most severe infections (AOM-SOS score > 8).
- There were no differences between the antibiotic and control groups with regard to the use of acetaminophen or the utilization of health care resources.

Table 13.1 SUMMARY OF THE TRIAL'S KEY FINDINGS

Outcome	Antibiotics Group	Control Group	P Value
Initial symptom resolution[a]			0.14[c]
Day 2	35%	28%	
Day 4	61%	54%	
Day 7	80%	74%	
Sustained symptom resolution[b]			0.04[c]
Day 2	20%	14%	
Day 4	41%	36%	
Day 7	67%	53%	
Symptom burden[d]	2.79	3.42	0.01
Clinical failure[e]			
At or before day 4–5	4%	23%	<0.001
At or before day 10–12	16%	51%	<0.001
Infection-related complications			
Mastoiditis	0%	1%	Nonsignificant[f]
Tympanic membrane perforation	1%	5%	Nonsignificant[f]
Antibiotic-related complications			
Diarrhea	25%	15%	0.05
Diaper rash	51%	35%	0.008
Oral thrush	5%	1%	Nonsignificant[f]

[a] Defined as AOM-SOS score of 0 or 1.
[b] Defined as two consecutive recordings of an AOM-SOS score of 0 or 1.
[c] For overall trend.
[d] Defined as the mean weighted AOM-SOS scores over first 7 days of follow-up.
[e] Defined at days 4–5 as a "lack of substantial improvement in symptoms, a worsening of signs on otoscopic examination, or both" and at days 10–12 as "the failure to achieve complete or nearly complete resolution of symptoms and otoscopic signs" with the exception of middle ear effusion.
[f] Actual P value not reported.

Criticisms and Limitations: The children in this study had acute otitis media diagnosed using stringent criteria. The findings are not applicable to children with an "uncertain" diagnosis of otitis media (e.g., those with no clear bulging of the tympanic membrane).

The authors defined clinical failure based (in part) on findings on otoscopic exam; however, it is uncertain whether children who become asymptomatic but have otoscopic findings of persistent middle-ear infection are at increased risk for recurrent symptomatic illness.

The authors chose amoxicillin-clavulanate for this study as it has been shown to be the most effective oral antibiotic for acute otitis media. Guidelines from the American Academy of Pediatrics and the American Academy of Family Practice recommend amoxicillin as first-line therapy, however.

Other Relevant Studies and Information:

- Other trials comparing immediate antibiotics with watchful waiting in children with acute otitis media have also generally suggested that antibiotics lead to modestly faster resolution of symptoms but increased rates of side effects (particularly diarrhea and rash).[2-5]
- Data on the impact of antibiotic therapy on antimicrobial resistance are limited; however, one study suggests that antibiotics lead to an increase in the rates of nasopharyngeal carriage of resistant *Streptococcus pneumoniae*.[6]
- Guidelines from the American Academy of Pediatrics and the American Academy of Family Practice recommend antibiotics in the following circumstances[7]:
  - all children <6 months with suspected otitis media
  - children 6 months–2 years when the symptoms are severe
  - children >2 years if the diagnosis is certain and the illness is severe

The guidelines state that watchful waiting with close observation may be considered for:

- children 6 months–2 years in whom the symptoms are not severe and the diagnosis is uncertain
- children >2 years in whom either the diagnosis is uncertain or the symptoms are not severe

Summary and Implications: Among children <2 years with stringently diagnosed acute otitis media, amoxicillin-clavulanate hastened the resolution of symptoms, reduced the overall symptom burden, and resulted in a lower rate of treatment failure but was associated with side effects (diarrhea and diaper dermatitis). Guidelines from the American Academy of Pediatrics (listed above) provide recommendations regarding which children with suspected acute otitis media should receive antibiotics versus watchful waiting with close observation.

CLINICAL CASE: ANTIBIOTICS FOR ACUTE OTITIS MEDIA

Case History:

An 18-month-old girl is brought to the office by her father with 36 hours of rhinorrhea, irritability, and a low grade fever (99.5°F). She has been eating normally, but awoke several times the previous night crying.

On exam, the girl is well-appearing with evidence of rhinorrhea and a temperature of 99.2°F. Otherwise her vital signs are within normal limits. You attempt to look in her ears but have difficulty making her stay still. From the brief look you get, it appears she may have a middle ear effusion in her right ear and perhaps a slightly erythematous tympanic membrane without bulging.

Based on the results of this trial, should you prescribe this girl an antibiotic for the treatment of acute otitis media?

Suggested Answer:

The above-described trial demonstrated that antibiotics are effective in children under 2 years of age with acute otitis media diagnosed using stringent criteria.

The girl in this vignette has an uncertain diagnosis of acute otitis media (her symptoms could be due entirely to a viral upper respiratory infection). In addition, her symptoms are relatively mild. Thus, the results of the trial do not necessarily apply to this patient.

Guidelines from the American Academy of Pediatrics and the American Academy of Family Practice indicate that watchful waiting with close observation—rather than immediate antibiotics—can be considered for children 6 months–2 years with an uncertain diagnosis of otitis media and mild symptoms. Thus, the girl in this vignette would be a good candidate for watchful waiting. If the watchful waiting strategy is chosen, the father should be instructed to call the office immediately should his daughter's condition worsen or not improve within a few days (if her condition worsens, she would likely need to be treated with antibiotics). Someone from the clinic might also call the family a couple of days later to make sure the girl is improving.

References

1. Hoberman A et al. Treatment of acute otitis media in children under 2 years of age. *N Engl J Med.* 2011;364(2):105–115.
2. Glasziou PP, Del Mar CB, Sanders SL, Hayem M. Antibiotics for acute otitis media in children. *Cochrane Database Syst Rev.* 2004;(1):CD000219.
3. Coker TR et al. Diagnosis, microbial epidemiology, and antibiotic treatment of acute otitis media in children: a systematic review. *JAMA.* 2010;304(19):2161.
4. Tähtinen PA et al. A placebo-controlled trial of antimicrobial treatment for acute otitis media. *N Engl J Med.* 2011;364(2):116–126.
5. Tähtinen PA et al. Delayed versus immediate antimicrobial treatment for acute otitis media. *Pediatr Infect Dis J.* 2012;31(12):1227–1232.
6. McCormick DP et al. Nonsevere acute otitis media: a clinical trial comparing outcomes of watchful waiting vs. immediate antibiotic treatment. *Pediatrics.* 2005;115(6):1455.
7. American Academy of Pediatrics Subcommittee on Management of Acute Otitis Media. Diagnosis and management of acute otitis media. *Pediatrics.* 2004;113(5):1451.

14

The Human Papillomavirus Vaccine

The Future II Trial

MICHAEL HOCHMAN, REVISED BY NINA SHAPIRO

In the Future II trial, [3.6% of] vaccinated women received [a diagnosis of grade 2 or 3 cervical intraepithelial neoplasia or adenocarcinoma in situ] over an average of 3 years, as compared with [4.4% of] unvaccinated women . . . [Still] a cautious approach may be warranted in light of important unanswered questions about overall vaccine effectiveness, duration of protection, and adverse effects that may emerge over time.

—Sawaya and Smith-Mccune[1]

Research Question: Is the quadrivalent human papillomavirus (HPV) vaccine against HPV types 6, 11, 16, and 18 safe and effective?[2]

- HPV-16 and HPV-18 cause 70% of all cervical cancers.
- HPV-6 and HPV-11 cause the majority of anogenital warts.

Funding: Merck

Year Study Began: 2002

Year Study Published: 2007

Study Location: 90 study sites in 13 countries in both the developed and developing world.

Who Was Studied: Girls and women 15–26 years old.

Who Was Excluded: Women who were pregnant, those who reported abnormal Papanicolaou (Pap) smear results at baseline, and those with >4 sexual partners.

How Many Patients: 12,167

Study Overview: See Figure 14.1 for a summary of the study design.

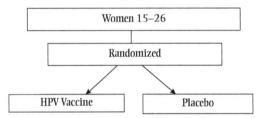

Figure 14.1 Summary of FUTURE II's Design.

Study Intervention: Women assigned to the HPV vaccine group received the vaccine upon enrollment, at 2 months, and at 6 months. Women assigned to the placebo group received a placebo injection according to the same schedule.

Women in both groups underwent Pap smears and anogenital swabs for HPV DNA testing at baseline and at 1, 6, 24, 36, and 48 months after the third vaccine (or placebo) injection.

Patients with abnormal Pap smears were managed according to standard protocols.

Follow-Up: A mean of 3 years.

Endpoints: Primary outcome: A composite of high-grade cervical lesions due to HPV-16 and HPV-18 including cervical intraepithelial neoplasia (CIN) grades 2 or 3, adenocarcinoma in situ, or invasive cervical cancer. Secondary outcome: High-grade cervical lesions due to any HPV type.

- CIN is a precancerous dysplastic lesion that is a precursor to squamous cell carcinoma of the cervix (the most common type of cervical cancer in the United States).
- CIN is graded on a scale of 1 to 3; CIN 1 is a low-grade lesion that frequently regresses and is managed with close monitoring; CIN 2

and CIN 3 are high-grade lesions that, if left untreated, often progress to invasive cancer.
- Adenocarcinoma in situ is another type of precancerous dysplastic lesion that may progress to adenocarcinoma (adenocarcinoma represents about 25% of cervical cancers in the United States).

RESULTS

- There were no cases of invasive cervical cancer during the study period in either group (see Table 14.1).
- Vaccine side effects appeared to be minor, though patients in the vaccine group did report slightly higher rates of injection site pain, seasonal allergies, and neck pain than patients in the placebo group.
- HPV vaccination did not appear to prevent the development of high-grade cervical lesions due to HPV-16 or HPV-18 among patients already infected with these HPV types at baseline.
- 99% of women who received the vaccine developed detectable levels of neutralizing HPV antibodies after vaccination. However, only 68% continued to have detectable antibody levels against the HPV-18 serotype at month 24.
- HPV vaccination lowered rates of high-grade lesions due to HPV-16 or HPV-18 as well as high-grade lesions due to any HPV type (see Table 14.1).

Table 14.1. SUMMARY OF FUTURE II's KEY FINDINGS[A]

Outcome	HPV Vaccine Group	Placebo Group	P Value[b]
High-grade lesions due to HPV-16 or HPV-18[c]	<0.1	0.3	Significant
High-grade lesions due to any HPV type[d]	1.3	1.5	Significant

[a] Rates are per 100 person-years, that is, the number of events that occurred for every 100 years of participant time. For example, 0.3 events per 100 person-years means that there were, on average, 0.3 events among 50 subjects who were each enrolled in the trial for 2 years.
[b] Actual P values not reported.
[c] Only includes patients who were negative for HPV-16 and HPV-18 at baseline and the 1-month postvaccination visit, and who closely followed the study protocol.
[d] Includes all enrolled patients, including those who had HPV-16 or HPV-18 at baseline and those who did not follow the study protocol closely. This analysis may better mimic "real-world" clinical practice.

Criticisms and Limitations: Although HPV vaccination led to a significant reduction in the rates of high-grade cervical lesions, the absolute reduction was modest ("129 women would need to be vaccinated in order to prevent one case of grade 2 or 3 cervical intraepithelial, neoplasia or adenocarcinoma in situ" during 3 years of follow-up[1]). Some experts have argued that this relatively small benefit does not justify HPV vaccination given the uncertainty about long-term vaccine safety and effectiveness.

HPV vaccination led to a reduction in precancerous cervical lesions but not a reduction in cervical cancer (cervical cancer rates are extremely low with effective cervical cancer screening). Because many precancerous lesions do not progress to cervical cancer, particularly with effective cervical cancer screening, the reduction in cancer rates from HPV vaccination is likely to be considerably smaller than the reduction in rates of precancerous lesions observed in this trial.

Although the clinical effectiveness of HPV vaccination did not appear to wane during the course of the study, only 68% of patients continued to have detectable antibody levels for the HPV-18 serotype at month 24. Follow-up data from Future II will be needed to determine whether the effectiveness of HPV vaccination persists beyond 3 years of follow-up.

Other Relevant Studies and Information:

- The Future I trial, which included fewer patients than Future II, showed that HPV vaccination led to a modest absolute reduction in composite rates of CIN 1, 2, and 3, and a modest absolute reduction in the rates of anogenital and vaginal warts.[3]
- The Patricia trial showed that a bivalent HPV vaccine against HPV-16 and HPV-18 was modestly effective in preventing CIN 2.
- Another trial showed that the quadrivalent HPV vaccine reduces the rates of HPV infection and the "development of related external genital lesions in males 16 to 26 years of age,"[4] as well as the rates of anal intraepithelial neoplasia (a precursor to anal cancer).[5]
- Following introduction of the HPV vaccine in 2006, the prevalence of HPV types included in the vaccine decreased from 11.5% to 5.1% among teenage females.[6]
- Both the quadrivalent and bivalent HPV vaccines have been approved in the United States and are recommended for girls 11–12 years of age and for girls and women ≤26 who did not receive the vaccine when they were younger; the quadrivalent vaccine has also been approved for use in males 9–26.

Summary and Implications: The quadrivalent HPV vaccine led to a modest absolute reduction in high-grade cervical lesions that are precursors to cervical cancer in girls and women 15–26. The vaccine is now recommended for adolescents and young adults of both sexes. Some experts remain cautious, however, because the absolute benefits of the vaccine are small and of uncertain duration, and may not justify yet unknown safety risks.

CLINICAL CASE: HUMAN PAPILLOMAVIRUS VACCINATION

Case History:
You are evaluating a 12 year-old girl during her routine annual check-up. When you mention to her that the Centers for Disease Control recommend HPV vaccination for 11- and 12-year-old girls, she appears apprehensive. She says, "I hate shots. Do I really need this vaccine?" Upon further questioning, the girl also tells you that she is not currently sexually active and does not plan on becoming sexually active in the near future.

What can you tell this girl about the risks and benefits of HPV vaccination based on the results of Future II?

Suggested Answer:
Future II demonstrated the effectiveness of the quadrivalent HPV vaccine in preventing high-grade cervical lesions that are precursors of cervical cancer. Girls and women are probably most likely to benefit from vaccination prior to the onset of sexual activity when they are at risk for acquiring HPV infections. As this girl's doctor, you might emphasize that although she is not planning on becoming sexually active in the near future, it is best for her to receive the vaccine before she does become sexually active.

On the other hand, the absolute benefits of the vaccine are relatively modest. In addition, we do not yet know whether there are any long-term safety concerns with the vaccine, or even if the vaccine will remain effective in preventing HPV infection in the long term.

You might handle this situation by recommending the vaccine to your patient (and her family), but inform her that it would also be reasonable to decline. Regardless of whether or not she decides to be vaccinated, your patient should receive regular Pap smears when she reaches the appropriate age (21 according to guidelines from the American College of Obstetrics and Gynecology).

References

1. Sawaya GF, Smith-McCune K. HPV vaccination—More answers, more questions. *N Engl J Med*. 2007;356:1991–1993.
2. The Future II Study Group. Quadrivalent vaccine against human papillomavirus to prevent high-grade cervical lesions. *N Engl J Med*. 2007;356:1915–1927.
3. Garland SM et al. Quadrivalent vaccine against human papillomavirus to prevent anogenital disease. *N Engl J Med*. 2007;356:1928.
4. Giuliano AR et al. Efficacy of quadrivalent HPV vaccine against HPV infection and disease in males. *N Engl J Med*. 2011;364(5):401.
5. Palefsky JM et al. HPV vaccine against anal HPV infection and anal intraepithelial neoplasia. *N Engl J Med*. 2011;365(17):1576–1585.
6. Markowitz LE et al. Reduction in human papillomavirus (HPV) prevalence among young women following HPV vaccine introduction in the United States, National Health and Nutrition Examination Surveys, 2003–2010. *J Infect Dis*. Epub 2013 Jun 19.

15

Evidence of Decrease in Vaccine-Type Human Papillomavirus (HPV) and Herd Protection in Adolescents and Young Women

NINA SHAPIRO

We found evidence of a substantial decrease in vaccine-type HPV prevalence in the community, as well as evidence of herd protection, only 4 years after the quadrivalent HPV vaccine was introduced; this is expected to translate into a decrease in cervical intraepithelial neoplasia (CIN) and ultimately cervical cancer in the community.

—KAHN ET AL.[1]

Research Question: What is the short-term impact of HPV vaccination on the prevalence of HPV in vaccinated women? Is there evidence of herd protection in unvaccinated women since the introduction of the HPV vaccine? Does vaccination increase the prevalence of other nonvaccine-type strains of the HPV virus?

Funding: National Institute of Allergy and Infectious Diseases (RO1 073713); National Institutes of Health (NIAID/NIH).

Year Study Began: 2006

Year Study Published: 2012

Study Location: Teen Health Center at Cincinnati Children's Hospital Medical Center and a community health center affiliated with the Cincinnati Health Department.

Who Was Studied: Young women 13–26 years of age who had engaged in sexual contact, defined as genital-oral or genital-genital contact with a male or female partner. The prevaccination surveillance study (2006–2007) enrolled only study participants who had not been previously vaccinated, whereas the postvaccination surveillance study (2009–2010) enrolled study participants who were either unvaccinated or who had received at least one HPV vaccine dose before study enrollment.

Who Was Excluded: Women who enrolled in the prevaccination surveillance study were excluded from participation in the postvaccination surveillance study.

How Many Patients: 368 women in the prevaccination surveillance study and 409 women in the postvaccination surveillance study.

Study Overview: See Figure 15.1 for a summary of the trial design.

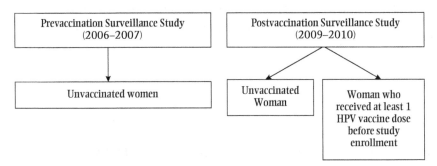

Figure 15.1 Summary of the Trial's Design.

Participant Testing: Cervicovaginal swabs were collected from all participants and genotyped to detect the presence of HPV subtypes. Participants completed self-administered questionnaires to assess demographic factors, HPV knowledge, gynecologic history, and sexual behaviors. The study authors controlled for significant differences between the vaccinated and unvaccinated groups, and selection bias, using a propensity score analysis.

Follow-Up: None.

Endpoints: The prevalence rates in the prevaccination and postvaccination surveillance studies of the following:

1. Any type of HPV infection
2. High-risk HPV—positive for ≥1 of the following HPV types: 16, 18, 26, 31, 33, 35, 39, 45, 51, 52, 53, 56, 58, 59, 67, 68, 70, 73, 82, and IS39
3. Vaccine-type HPV—positive for ≥1 of the following HPV types: 6, 11, 16, and/or 18
4. High-risk, vaccine-type HPV—positive for HPV 16 and/or 18
5. Nonvaccine-type HPV—positive for ≥1 HPV type other than 6, 11, 16, and/or 18
6. High-risk, nonvaccine-type HPV—positive for ≥1 high-risk HPV type other than 6, 11, 16, and/or 18

RESULTS

- Overall prevalence of HPV (all types of HPV) in all study participants increased by 8.5% between the prevaccination and postvaccination surveillance studies.
- The absolute decrease in the prevalence of vaccine-type HPV was 18.3% between the prevaccination and postvaccination surveillance studies for all study participants, both vaccinated and unvaccinated, demonstrating the effect of the introduction of the HPV vaccine in this community. Perhaps of even more significance, the overall prevalence of vaccine-type HPV decreased by 57.7%.
  - The prevalence of vaccine-type HPV decreased 21.9% (overall prevalence decreased by 68.9%) in the vaccinated participants.
  - The prevalence of vaccine-type HPV decreased 14.8% (overall prevalence decreased by 49.0%) in the unvaccinated participants, and similar changes were noted for high-risk, vaccine-type HPV, providing evidence for herd protection.
- The prevalence of nonvaccine type HPV increased by 14.0% and the prevalence of high-risk, nonvaccine-type HPV increased by 7.6% for all study participants, although these were only statistically significant for the vaccinated participants.

Criticisms and Limitations: The study sample primarily included minority, low-income, young women, a specific subset of the population that is at increased risk for HPV infection, and therefore the results may not reflect the general population. In addition, women >12 years of age, considered to be part of the "catch-up" age group, were included in this study; however, the group mainly targeted for vaccination are 11- to 12-year-old girls. The authors also attempted to correct for a number of variables that statistically differed between the study samples, but these confounders still might have impacted the differences in HPV prevalence found between the study groups. Finally, the increase in prevalence of nonvaccine-type HPV was found to be significantly increased in vaccinated participants.

While type-replacement is unlikely to be caused by vaccine administration, and individual HPV types behave independently of one another, larger long-term studies are needed to further address this critical issue. If vaccination leads to an increase in high-risk nonvaccine-type HPV, it would undermine the utility of HPV vaccination.

Other Relevant Studies and Information:

- Recommendations of the American Academy of Pediatrics[2]:
  - Girls 11–12 years of age should be immunized routinely with 3 doses of HPV4 or HPV2. The vaccines can be administered starting at 9 years of age.
  - All girls and women 13–26 years of age who have not been immunized previously or have not completed the full vaccine series should also be vaccinated.
  - Boys 11–12 years of age should be immunized routinely with 3 doses of HPV4. The vaccine can be given starting at 9 years of age at the discretion of the physician.
  - All boys and men 13–21 years of age who have not been immunized previously or have not completed the full vaccine series, as well as all men 22–26 years of age at high risk for HPV, should receive HPV4 vaccine.
  - In 2012, only 33% of teenage girls ages 13–17 years had received 3 doses of HPV vaccine.[3]

Summary and Implications: This analysis demonstrated that HPV vaccination reduces the prevalence of vaccine-type HPV infection both among women who did and did not receive the HPV vaccine. The reduction in HPV prevalence among unvaccinated women is presumably the result of herd protection. These findings support recommendations for vaccinating adolescents and young adults.

CLINICAL CASE: VACCINE-TYPE HUMAN PAPILLOMAVIRUS AND EVIDENCE OF HERD PROTECTION AFTER VACCINE INTRODUCTION

Case History:

A 16-year-old sexually active female who is not vaccinated with the human papillomavirus quadrivalent vaccine (HPV4) comes in for gynecologic examination. Although it is likely that she has had exposure to the human papillomavirus, do you recommend that this individual receive the HPV4 vaccine?

Suggested Answer:

It is possible that this young woman has attained a degree of herd immunity, depending on the community of sexual partners with whom she has been in contact. It is recommended that she receive the HPV4 vaccine.

References

1. Kahn JA, Brown DR, Ding L, et al. Vaccine-type human papillomavirus and evidence of herd protection after vaccine introduction. *Pediatrics.* 2012;130(2):e249–e256.
2. Committee on Infectious Diseases. HPV vaccine recommendations. *Pediatrics.* 2012;129(3):602–605.
3. Human papillomavirus vaccination coverage among adolescent girls, 2007–2012, and postlicensure vaccine safety monitoring, 2006–2013—United States. *MMWR.* 2013:62(29):591–595.

16

Effects of Lead Exposure in Childhood

ASHAUNTA ANDERSON

*In this extended follow-up study, in which the mean length of follow-up was
11.1 years, we found that the associations reported earlier between lead and
children's academic progress and cognitive functioning persisted into young
adulthood.*

— NEEDLEMAN ET AL.[1]

Research Question: Do the negative neurobehavioral effects of low-level lead
exposure during childhood persist into adulthood?[1]

Funding: Not reported.

Year Study Began: 1975

Year Study Published: 1990

Study Location: Chelsea and Somerville, Massachusetts school systems.

Who Was Studied: First- and second-grade students from English-speaking
homes with initial dentin lead levels <6 ppm or >24 ppm.

Who Was Excluded: Initially, the investigators excluded those who were not discharged from the hospital at the same time as their mothers after birth, who had a significant head injury, who had a history of lead toxicity, or whose dentin lead levels did not meet predefined criteria. Follow-up analyses showed that these factors did not affect the outcomes of interest, so the initially excluded children were included in this analysis.

How Many Patients: 132

Study Overview: See Figure 16.1 for a summary of the study design.

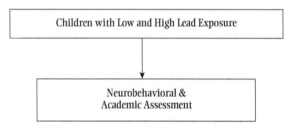

Figure 16.1 Summary of the Study's Design.

Follow-Up: Children who participated in the original study at ages 6 and 7 years old[2] were recontacted an average of 11.1 years later. Subjects were identified for reevaluation using available telephone directories, driver's license records, and other local records. Participants were an average of 18.4 years old at the time of reevaluation.

Study Intervention: Neurobehavioral testing was performed for all participants by an evaluator blinded to initial lead exposure level. Participants also completed a number of cognitive assessments and scales on antisocial behavior and violent crimes. For students beyond 11th grade, investigators collected school records on class size and rank, highest grade completed, and number of days absent and tardy in the last full semester.

Endpoints: Markers of neurobehavioral, cognitive, and school performance; and markers of delinquency.

RESULTS

- Childhood exposure to lead was associated with 7-fold increased odds of failure to graduate from high school; lower class standing; greater absenteeism; reading disabilities; and deficits in vocabulary, fine motor skills, reaction time, and hand-eye coordination (see Table 16.1).
  - A dose-dependent relationship was observed between increasing dentin lead level and both increasing reading disabilities and worsening high school graduation rates.
- Comparison of children with dentin lead levels <10 ppm to those with lead levels >10 ppm predicted failure to graduate from high school with a sensitivity of 0.71 (± SE 0.12) and a specificity of 0.61 (± SE 0.05)

Table 16.1. REGRESSION OF YOUNG ADULTHOOD OUTCOMES
ON CHILDHOOD DENTIN LEAD LEVELS

Outcome	Parameter Estimate	Standard Error	P Value
Highest grade achieved	−0.027	0.01	0.013
Reading grade equivalent	−0.072	0.021	0.001
Class standing	−0.006	0.003	0.048
Absence from school[a]	4.73	1.8	0.01
Grammatical reasoning	0.178	0.068	0.011
Vocabulary	−0.122	0.033	0.001
Finger tapping	−0.133	0.05	0.01
Hand-eye coordination	0.048	0.019	0.01
Reaction time[a]	12.9	6.3	0.042
Preferred hand	10.3	5.5	0.06
Non-preferred hand	−0.739	0.35	0.038
Minor antisocial behavior[a]			

Adapted from Table 3 of the original study, which reports the multiple regression analysis controlling for age, sex, birth order, family size, mother's age at the participant's birth, length of the neonatal stay in the hospital, maternal education level, maternal IQ, socioeconomic status, and current alcohol use:
Needleman et al. The long-term effects of exposure to low doses of lead in childhood. *N Engl J Med.* 1990; 322:83–88.
[a] The main effect was the natural log of the mean dentin lead level.

Criticisms and Limitations: Although the study controlled for several covariates, some uncontrolled confounding variables may remain because it was not a randomized controlled trial. It is also important to note that the subset of original participants available for this reevaluation were not representative of the original sample. The retested participants had lower dentin lead levels, higher socioeconomic status, and better academic standing, among other differences. The association between dentin lead level and IQ was less strong in the retested group, but statistically similar to that of the original group. This biases the studies results toward the null.

Other Relevant Studies and Information:

- Meta-analyses of the literature consistently demonstrate a negative effect of lead—even low lead levels—on academic outcomes,[3] including a 1- to 2.6-point drop in IQ for an increase in blood lead from 10 to 20 mcg/dL.[4,5]
- Behavioral problems have also been linked to childhood lead exposure:
  - Preschoolers with low-level lead exposure (10–24 mcg/dL blood lead) had more behavioral problems than those with no exposure (<10 mcg/dL).[6]
  - 11-year-old boys with higher bone lead levels had more antisocial and delinquent behavior.[7]
- Low-level lead exposure during the prenatal and neonatal periods may exert a negative effect on infant neurobehavioral development.[8]
- According to a policy statement of the American Academy of Pediatrics, even blood lead concentrations lower than 10 mcg/dL may adversely affect cognition, so it is best to screen child lead levels at age 1 year and again at the typical peak exposure at 2 years of age.[9]

Summary and Implications: Childhood exposure to lead, even at low levels without symptoms, had important long-lasting negative effects on behavioral and academic outcomes. Clinicians and public health officials are alerted to the importance of detecting and preventing lead toxicity early in life.

CLINICAL CASE: EFFECTS OF LEAD EXPOSURE IN CHILDHOOD

Case History:
A 2-year-old boy presents to the clinic for a well child visit. He has no significant medical history and no acute complaints. He eats a varied diet and has no elimination issues. According to his parents, he can kick a ball, feed himself, use two-word phrases, and follow two-part commands.

On examination, his growth parameters are normal for age and gender. Vital signs are within normal limits. He is cooperative and interactive. You are able to understand roughly half of what he says. He shows off his ability to run and hold a pen. The rest of his exam is unremarkable.

You explain to the boy's parents that today he will need to have the lead level checked in his blood. The parents were looking forward to a visit free of needle sticks and ask for more information on why this particular test is recommended.

Suggested Answer:
You begin by describing the normal mouthing behavior of children 6 months to 3 years of age. Even though lead has been removed from most paints and gasoline, it can still be present in dust and other forms that may not be readily visible to the naked eye. In most places like the United States, blood lead levels will peak at 2 years of age, the age of their son. In the best situation, the boy would have already had his blood lead level checked at 1 year of age to catch any elevated levels prior to peak levels. It is now important to make sure the level is not too high, so he does not experience preventable nervous system problems. Studies have shown that high levels of lead are linked to lower IQ, more behavioral problems, and delayed development. Today, their son shows none of these problems, and checking his blood lead level helps keep it that way. If it turns out that his lead level is too high, you would be able to take the necessary steps to lower it to a safe level.

References

1. Needleman et al. The long-term effects of exposure to low doses of lead in childhood. *N Engl J Med.* 1990;322:83–88.
2. Needleman et al. Deficits in psychologic and classroom performance of children with elevated dentine lead levels. *N Engl J Med.* 1979; 300:689–695.
3. Needleman HL et al. Low-level lead exposure and the IQ of children: A meta-analysis of modern studies. *JAMA.* 1990;263:673–678.

4. Schwartz J. Low-level lead exposure and children's IQ: Meta-analysis and search for a threshold. *Environ Res.* 1994;65(1):42–55.

5. Pocock SJ et al. Environmental lead and children's intelligence: A systematic review of the epidemiological evidence. *BMJ.* 1994;309(6963):1189–1197.

6. Mendelsohn AL et al. Low-level lead exposure and behavior in early childhood. *Pediatrics.* 1998;101(3):E10.

7. Needleman HL et al. Bone lead levels and delinquent behavior. *JAMA.* 1996;275(5):363–369.

8. Dietrich KN et al. Low-level fetal lead exposure effect on neurobehavioral development in early infancy. *Pediatrics.* 1987;80(5):721–730.

9. American Academy of Pediatrics Committee on Environmental Health. Lead exposure in children: Prevention, detection, and management. *Pediatrics.* 2005;116(4):1036–1046.

SECTION 8

Hematology

17

Iron Supplementation for Breastfed Infants

ASHAUNTA ANDERSON

Iron supplementation of breast-fed infants appears safe and might have beneficial hematologic and developmental effects for some infants.

—FRIEL ET AL.[1]

Research Question: Does early iron supplementation affect the hematologic and neurodevelopmental status of healthy, breastfed infants?[1]

Funding: Canadian Institutes of Health Research.

Year Study Began: 1999

Year Study Published: 2003

Study Location: Postpartum unit and clinics in St. John's, Newfoundland.

Who Was Studied: Infants of parents planning to exclusively breastfeed, meaning no more than one supplemental feeding per day for a minimum of 4 months.

Who Was Excluded: Gestational age <37 weeks, birth weight <2.5 kg, multiple pregnancy, admission to the intensive care unit, or significant congenital anomaly

How Many Patients: 77

Study Overview: See Figure 17.1 for a summary of the study design.

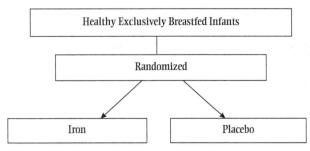

Figure 17.1 Summary of the Trial's Design.

Follow-Up: Children were followed from 1 month up to 18 months of age.

Study Intervention: Infants successfully breastfeeding at age 1 month were randomized to receive ferrous sulfate 7.5 mg of elemental iron daily or placebo (similarly flavored syrup with no medication) for 5 months. Parents and investigators were blinded to the assignment of iron versus placebo. A nurse was available to answer questions about study medications and breastfeeding.

Endpoints: Blood draws were performed during clinic visits at ages 1, 3.5, 6, and 12 months to assess hemoglobin, mean corpuscular volume, hematocrit, red blood cell superoxide dismutase, catalase, ferritin, and plasma levels of ferric-reducing antioxidant power, copper, and zinc. Weight, length, head circumference, and dietary histories were also assessed at each clinic visit. At a later visit between 12 and 18 months, development and visual acuity were assessed using the mental and psychomotor indexes of the Bayley Scales and Teller visual acuity cards.

RESULTS

- When the iron group was compared to the placebo group:
  - Dropout rates, duration of therapy, gastrointestinal symptoms, and minor illnesses were similar.
  - Iron levels remained higher in the iron group until 12 months of age when all infants had stopped breastfeeding.
  - Weight, length, and head circumference were similar at every clinic visit.

- Levels of superoxide dismutase, catalase, plasma ferric-reducing antioxidant power, copper, and zinc were similar at every visit.
- Mean corpuscular volume at 3.5 and 6 months of age and hemoglobin at 6 months of age were higher in the iron group.
- Trends suggested that infants in the iron group were relatively protected from iron deficiency and iron deficiency anemia (see Table 17.1).
- Infants in the iron group performed an average of 7 points higher on the psychomotor developmental indexes, but outcomes were not different for the mental developmental indexes (intention to treat analysis).
- Infants in the iron group showed better visual acuity, but only when noncompliers were excluded.

Table 17.1. EFFECTS OF SUPPLEMENTAL IRON
ON DEVELOPMENT AND VISUAL ACUITY[a]

	Iron Group	Placebo Group
Mental Developmental Indexes[b] Intention to treat	108 ± 8.0 (26)	108 ± 10.4 (20)
Mental Developmental Indexes >30 days of iron	109 ± 7.6 (24)	108 ± 10.8 (17)
Psychomotor Developmental Indexes[c] Intention to treat	100 ± 12 (26)[d]	93 ± 8.8 (20)
Psychomotor Developmental Indexes >30 days of iron	100 ± 11.8 (24)[d]	92 ± 8.2 (17)
Visual acuity Intention to treat	1.43 ± 1.20 (25)	0.91 ± 1.13 (20)
Visual acuity >30 days of iron	1.54 ± 1.18 (23)[d]	0.87 ± 0.79 (17)

Adapted from Table III of the original study: Friel et al. A double-masked, randomized control trial of iron supplementation in early infancy in healthy term breast-fed infants. *J Pediatr.* 2003;143:582–586.
[a]Values are expressed as the sample mean Z score ± standard deviation, number of infants in parentheses.
[b]Bayley Mental Developmental Indexes.
[c]Bayley Psychomotor Developmental Indexes.
[d]$P < 0.05$.

Criticisms and Limitations: The authors originally intended to recruit 100 infants into each arm of the study in order to detect a 5% difference on the developmental indexes using standard power and alpha values. Inadequate funding limited recruitment to the 77 studied infants. Only 44 of the original 77 infants were present for the blood draw at 12 months of age, and 46 were available for the developmental assessment. Beyond attendance drop-off, consistent exclusive breastfeeding was difficult to ensure. It is possible that more robust results may have been attained with a larger sample size and improved compliance.

Other Relevant Studies and Information:

- In a randomized, placebo-controlled trial of 7 mg/day ferrous sulfate in breastfed infants 1–5 months old, iron status transiently improved, and no deleterious effects on growth were noted.[2]
- Systematic review of iron supplementation for iron deficiency anemia in children aged 6–24 months revealed improvement in hematologic measures with no consistent evidence for improved growth, development, or anemia.[3]
- The American Academy of Pediatrics Committee on Nutrition recommends the following approach to iron supplementation in breastfed infants.[4]
  - Healthy, term exclusively breastfed infants should receive 1 mg/kg daily oral iron from 4 months of age until complementary foods containing iron are started
    - The same recommendation applies to healthy, term infants who are receiving supplemental iron-enriched formula as long as more than half their daily feedings come from breast milk and they are not receiving complementary foods.
  - Preterm exclusively breastfed infants should receive 2 mg/kg daily supplemental iron by 1 month until iron-containing formula or complementary foods are started.
- Controversy remains regarding the benefits and safety of iron supplementation in healthy, term, exclusively breastfeeding infants.[5]

Summary and Implications: Supplemental iron in healthy, breastfed infants was associated with improved red blood cell indices at certain ages, psychomotor development, and visual acuity. Clinical utility is not clear for all the improvements, but it appears iron supplementation may protect a subset of breastfed infants from the usual decline in hemoglobin in early infancy and the associated neurodevelopmental sequelae. The American Academy of Pediatrics recommends iron supplementation for breastfed infants beginning at 4 months. However, in practice, these guidelines are not often followed due to the lack of proven clinical benefit of such supplementation.

CLINICAL CASE: IRON SUPPLEMENTATION FOR BREASTFED INFANTS

Case History:

A 5-month-old previously term girl comes to the county clinic for a physical examination. Her mother also asks you to fill out a form for the Women, Infants, and Children program. She admits that it has been hard to make ends meet lately, but her daughter appears to be growing well and starting to roll over on her own. The girl has no history of significant medical problems and is exclusively breastfed. She feeds and voids regularly. She has been tolerating her vitamin D drops with no issues. Her mother has no concerns about her health.

Upon examination, the girl is active and cooperative. She appears well-developed and well-nourished. All vital signs are unremarkable as is the rest of the physical examination.

You explain to the girl's mother that she missed the vaccines typically given to babies when they are 4 months old, but can have those in the clinic today. You also encourage her to continue taking daily vitamin D. The girl's mother points to a pamphlet she read in the waiting room and asks if her exclusively breastfed daughter also needs to receive daily iron to stay healthy.

Suggested Answer:

According to recommendations of the American Academy of Pediatrics Committee on Nutrition,[4] this girl is a good candidate for daily oral iron supplementation. She is exclusively breastfed and therefore receiving no additional food or formula, which may provide a source of iron. She has passed the age of 4 months when infants are at greater risk for iron deficiency anemia. The focal study of this chapter suggests that iron supplementation will lead to enhanced iron levels, psychomotor development, and visual acuity without significant side effects. This information may be relayed to the girl's mother with the caveat that other important outcomes have not been evaluated.

It is also important to take into consideration any risk factors each child may have for iron deficiency anemia, as it has been shown that iron deficiency with or without anemia has been linked to impaired neurodevelopment. Certainly, children who are born preterm, low birth weight, or otherwise predisposed to low iron stores are good candidates for iron supplementation while exclusively breastfeeding.[6] In addition, there is increased risk for iron deficiency in those with low socioeconomic backgrounds, Mexican American heritage, lead exposure, or special health care problems that inhibit proper feeding and growth.[6] The girl in this clinical case is eligible for means-tested nutritional support through WIC, which indicates a low socioeconomic status as a risk factor for iron deficiency. Therefore, she should receive daily oral iron supplementation until her diet includes iron-rich complementary foods.

References

1. Friel et al. A double-masked, randomized control trial of iron supplementation in early infancy in healthy term breast-fed infants. *J Pediatr.* 2003;143:582–586.
2. Ziegler et al. Iron supplementation of breastfed infants from an early age. *Am J Clin Nutr.* 2009;89:525–532.
3. McDonagh et al. Screening and routine supplementation for iron deficiency anemia: A systematic review. *Pediatrics.* 2015;135(4):723–733.
4. Baker et al. Clinical report—Diagnosis and prevention of iron deficiency and iron-deficiency anemia in infants and young children (0–3 years of age). *Pediatrics.* 2010;126:1040–1050.
5. Schanler et al. Concerns with early universal iron supplementation of breastfeeding infants. *Pediatrics.* 2011;127:e1097.
6. American Academy of Pediatrics Section on Breastfeeding. Breastfeeding and the use of human milk. *Pediatrics.* 2005;115:496–506.

Transfusion Strategies for Patients in Pediatric Intensive Care Units

JEREMIAH DAVIS

> ... a restrictive transfusion strategy can safely decrease the rate of exposure
> to red cells as well as the total number of transfusions in critically ill children.
> —LACROIX ET AL.[1]

Research Question: At what hemoglobin threshold should critically ill children be transfused?[1]

Funding: Canadian Institutes of Health Research and Fonds de la Recherche en Santé du Québec. In addition, three study authors received private industry funding and one was employed by the Canadian Blood Services.

Year Study Began: 2001

Year Study Published: 2007

Study Location: 19 tertiary-care pediatric intensive care units (ICUs) in four countries (Belgium, Canada, United Kingdom, and United States).

Who Was Studied: Children 3 days to 14 years old in pediatric ICUs meeting the following requirements:

- One or more hemoglobin concentrations of 9.5 g/dL or less within 7 days of admission to the ICU
- Mean systemic arterial pressure not less than 2 standard deviations below the normal mean for age
- Vasoactive infusions had not been increased for at least 2 hours prior to enrollment

Who Was Excluded: Children who were expected to stay in the ICU < 24 hours, those not approved by attending physician for participation, those <3 days or >14 years of age, those who were hemodynamically unstable, those <3 kg in weight, those never discharged from a neonatal ICU, or those already enrolled in a different study were excluded. Also excluded were subjects with acute blood loss, cardiovascular problems, hemolysis or low platelet counts, hypoxemia, care withheld or withdrawn, predicted survival <24 hours, brain death, or required invasive exchange therapies (plasmapheresis, extracorporeal membrane oxygenation, etc.). Finally, any individual who was unable to receive blood products or was pregnant could not participate in the study.

How Many Patients: 637

Study Overview: See Figure 18.1 for a summary of the trial design.

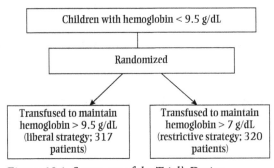

Figure 18.1 Summary of the Trial's Design.

Study Intervention: Children assigned to the restrictive-strategy group were transfused with leukocyte-reduced packed red blood cells (PRBCs) within 12 hours of a recorded hemoglobin concentration below 7 g/dL; this group was transfused to a target range of 8.5–9.5 g/dL. Those in the liberal-strategy group were transfused with leukocyte-reduced PRBCs within 12 hours of a recorded hemoglobin below 9.5 g/dL with a target range of 11–12 g/dL. Subjects were followed for up to 28 ICU days or until time of death.

Follow-Up: 28 days maximum.

Endpoints: Primary outcomes: Proportion of patients who died during the 28-day period; concurrent dysfunction of two or more organ systems (multiple-organ-dysfunction syndrome, or MODS); or progression of MODS. Secondary outcomes: daily scores of the Pediatric Logistic Organ Dysfunction (PELOD) assessment; sepsis; transfusion reactions; nosocomial respiratory infections; adverse events; catheter-related infections; length of stay in the ICU and hospital; and mortality.

RESULTS

- At baseline, the mean hemoglobin concentration was similar between both groups (8.0 ± 1.0 g/dL vs. 8.0 ± 0.9 g/dL).
- Children in the liberal-strategy group received their first transfusions earlier than in the restrictive group: 0.1 days vs. 1.7 days, respectively.
- Those in the liberal-strategy group received first transfusions at lower hemoglobin concentrations than restrictive-strategy participants (8.1 ± 0.1 g/dL vs. 6.7 ± 0.5 g/dL, respectively).
- Hemoglobin was maintained above threshold more then 94% of the time.
- Children in the liberal-strategy group received more transfusions than those in the restrictive-strategy group (see Table 18.1).
- Rates of the major primary and secondary outcomes were similar between the two groups (see Table 18.1).

Table 18.1. SUMMARY OF THE TRIAL'S KEY FINDINGS

Outcome	Restrictive-Strategy	Liberal-Strategy	P Value
Total number of transfusions	301	542	<0.001
Percentage of patients receiving no transfusions	54%	2%	<0.001
Average number of transfusions per patient	0.9 ± 2.6	1.7 ± 2.2	<0.001
Percentage of patients with new or progressive MODS	12%	12%	Noninferior
Death from any cause during 28-day study	4%	4%	0.98
Nosocomial infections	20%	25%	0.16
At least one adverse event	30%	28%	0.59
Reactions to red-cell transfusions	1%	2%	0.34
Days of mechanical ventilation	6.2 ± 5.9	6.0 ± 5.4	0.76
Days of ICU stay after randomization	9.5 ± 7.9	9.9 ± 7.4	0.39

Criticisms and Limitations: This study examined relatively stable children in the ICU, but excluded 81% of children with hemoglobin levels <9.5 g/dL (see exclusion criteria above). Thus these findings only apply to a minority of pediatric ICU patients; however, they have important implications regarding the risk:benefit ratio of transfusion decisions.

Additionally, the protocol was suspended temporarily for 39 children (36 of whom received transfusions) in the restrictive-strategy group, and for 20 (11 of whom received transfusions) in the liberal-strategy group. During these suspensions, 71 and 61 transfusions, respectively, were administered. While this only affected a small portion (12% and 6%, respectively) of each group, in the restrictive-strategy group they accounted for 23% of all transfusions received. This may have affected the outcomes in these patients.

Other Relevant Studies and Information:

- Lacroix's study was the first of its kind in pediatrics. Since publication, there have been several post-hoc analyses performed:
  - Postoperative ICU patients[2] had similar outcomes between liberal and restrictive groups, but the restrictive group had a statistically significant shorter length of stay (7.7 ± 6.6 days vs. 11.6 ± 10.2 days).
  - Septic ICU patients had no significant differences in MODS or other outcomes.[3]

Summary and Implications: Critically ill pediatric patients 3 days to 14 years old, over 3 kg in weight and who are hemodynamically stable, have similar outcomes with a liberal transfusion strategy (transfusion target >9.5 g/dL) versus a restrictive transfusion strategy (transfusion target >7 g/dL). A restrictive strategy is associated with exposure to fewer blood products.

CLINICAL CASE: TRANSFUSION IN THE PEDIATRIC ICU

Case History:
An 11-year-old male is admitted into the Pediatric ICU after a noncontrast head CT obtained for acute ataxia reveals a posterior fossa mass. Your neurosurgical colleagues successfully decompressed the tumor and obtained tissue samples for analysis by pathology. The patient arrives to the unit intubated and sedated; his vital signs reveal tachycardia with heart rates in the 110 range. His blood pressure is stable with systolics in the 110 range and diastolics in the low 70s. Initial evaluation demonstrates an arterial blood gas (while ventilated) of pH 7.39 and CO_2 41, a normal white blood cell count, a hemoglobin concentration of 8.4 g/dL, and normal electrolytes postoperatively. The transferring anesthesiologist remarks, "He's kind of tachycardic postoperatively—he could probably use a transfusion to make him feel better."

Based on the results of this trial, should you transfuse this patient with PRBCs?

Suggested Answer:
The above-described trial demonstrated that compared to a liberal transfusion policy, a restrictive transfusion strategy using a hemoglobin concentration of 7 g/dL as a cutoff value resulted in similar outcomes for pediatric ICU patients such as this one. With a newly diagnosed brain tumor this patient likely will have a prolonged ICU stay while his recovery of function (and ability to oxygenate/ventilate) becomes more clear. He is hemodynamically stable and otherwise fits the same characteristics that the Lacroix study group demonstrated. He would be an optimal candidate for delaying transfusions until absolutely necessary—either due to a clinical change such as acute hemorrhage, or when his hemoglobin falls below 7 g/dL. Based on Lacroix's findings, his likelihood of multiple organ dysfunction or mortality is not increased by waiting, but the volume of PRBCs transfused will be less.

References

1. Lacroix J et al. Transfusion strategies for patients in pediatric intensive care units. N Eng J Med. 2007;356(16):1609–1619.
2. Rouette J et al. Red blood cell transfusion threshold in postsurgical pediatric intensive care patients: a randomized clinical trial. Ann Surg. 2010;251(3):421–427.
3. Karam O et al. Red blood cell transfusion thresholds in pediatric patients with sepsis. Ped Crit Care Med. 2011;12(5):512–518.

19

Prophylactic Penicillin in Sickle Cell Anemia

ASHAUNTA ANDERSON

This randomized, double-blind, multi-center trial demonstrated the effectiveness of prophylaxis with oral penicillin in significantly decreasing the incidence of pneumococcal septicemia in children with sickle cell anemia.
—GASTON ET AL.[1]

Research Question: Does daily oral penicillin decrease the incidence of severe infection due to *Streptococcus pneumoniae* in young children with sickle cell anemia?[1]

Funding: Penicillin donated by Wyeth Laboratories.

Year Study Began: 1983

Year Study Published: 1986

Study Location: 23 clinical sites.

Who Was Studied: Children 3–36 months of age with an SS hemoglobin pattern on electrophoresis.

Who Was Excluded: Children with a known penicillin allergy and those already on a long-term antibiotic or transfusion regimen.

How Many Patients: 215

Study Overview: See Figure 19.1 for a summary of the study design.

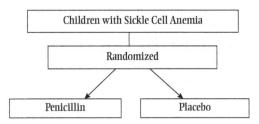

Figure 19.1 Summary of the Trial's Design.

Follow-Up: Children were followed for an average of 15 months. The trial was terminated 8 months early upon the recommendation of an independent advisory board.

Study Intervention: Children were randomized to 125 mg of oral penicillin V potassium twice daily or placebo (50 mg vitamin C twice daily). Parents and staff at the clinical sites were blinded to assignment. Approximately every 3 months, a history (including febrile events), physical examination, complete blood count, pill count, and test of urine penicillin levels were conducted. An additional urine penicillin level was collected by parents and submitted for analysis between regular clinic visits. At study entry and exit, nasopharyngeal culture and serum pneumococcal antibody titers were obtained.

When a serious bacterial infection was suspected, protocol-specified cultures were obtained and urine penicillin concentration was assessed. If *S. pneumoniae* was recovered by culture, the organism was serotyped and serum pneumococcal antibody was measured. For febrile illnesses requiring antibiotic administration, the study drug was discontinued and restarted upon completion of the antibiotic course. After the start of the trial, investigators decided to standardize the schedule of pneumococcal vaccination across the participating clinical sites.

Endpoints: Primary outcome: Documented severe infection caused by *S. pneumoniae*. Secondary outcome: Documented severe infection caused by any other organism. Documentation included clinical and laboratory evidence consistent with bacterial infection and recovery of an organism from the relevant body fluid. Severe infections included bacteremia, meningitis, and pneumonia that required hospitalization.

RESULTS

- Of the 15 cases of documented pneumococcal septicemia, 2 occurred
  in the penicillin group (n = 105) and 13 in the control group (n = 110;
  $P = 0.0025$) (see Figure 19.2).
  - Adjustment for risk factors did not change these findings.
  - Septicemia was the only type of severe pneumococcal infection
    documented.
- The 1-year incidence of pneumococcal septicemia was 0.02 in the
  penicillin group and 0.09 in the placebo group.
- Pneumococcal septicemia resulted in no deaths in the penicillin
  group, but 3 deaths in the placebo group, all of whom had received
  pneumococcal vaccine.
- One child in the penicillin group and 2 children in the placebo group
  developed *Haemophilus influenzae* type b septicemia, leading to the
  death of 1 child from the placebo group.
- Vaccine for *H. influenzae* type b was not available until late in the study.

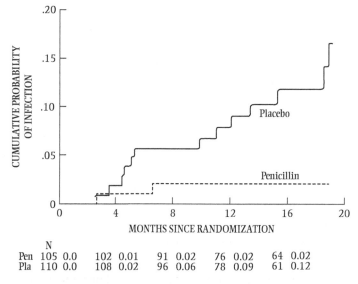

	N									
Pen	105	0.0	102	0.01	91	0.02	76	0.02	64	0.02
Pla	110	0.0	108	0.02	96	0.06	78	0.09	61	0.12

Figure 19.2 Cumulative Infection Rates for All Patients in the Prophylactic Penicillin
Study. Reprinted with permission from Gaston et al. "Prophylaxis with oral penicillin
in children with sickle cell anemia." *N Engl J Med*. 1986; 314:1593–1599.

Criticisms and Limitations: Although the investigators used two different
methods to measure medication compliance—pill counts and urine penicillin levels—patients ultimately provided an insufficient amount of data to allow
analysis. For this reason, they were unable to comment on the extent to which

patients in the penicillin or placebo groups consistently took their assigned medication. However, the likelihood is that children in the penicillin group did not maintain perfect fidelity to twice daily penicillin, and those in the placebo group did not receive long-term courses of penicillin. If perfect compliance could have been guaranteed, the investigators may have reported an even stronger prophylactic effect.

Other Relevant Studies and Information:

- Systematic review of 3 trials confirmed the protective effect of prophylactic penicillin against pneumococcal infection in young children with sickle cell disease (both homozygous SS and $S\beta_0$-thalassemia types).[2]
- In a randomized, double-blind, placebo-controlled trial of prophylactic penicillin discontinuation at age 5 years among children with sickle cell disease (SS and $S\beta_0$-thalassemia), no significant increased risk of severe pneumococcal infection was associated with discontinuation.[3]
- An expert panel outlined the management of sickle cell disease with the following strong recommendations:[4]
  - For children with sickle cell anemia (hemoglobin SS)
    - Oral prophylactic penicillin (125 mg for children <3 years of age and 250 mg for those ≥3 years) twice daily until age 5 years.
    - Annual transcranial Doppler screening from ages 2 to at least 16 years (measures the velocity of arterial blood flow in the brain).
    - Referral to long-term transfusion specialist if Doppler results are borderline (170–199 cm/s) or elevated (≥200 cm/s) to help prevent stroke.[5,6]
    - Hydroxyurea for children ≥9 months of age to help prevent disease-specific complications.[7,8]
  - For children with sickle cell disease (all genotypes)
    - Vaccination with the conjugate 13-valent pneumococcal vaccine (add 23-valent polysaccharide vaccine for those 19 years or older with asplenia).
    - Screening by ophthalmology for retinopathy by 10 years of age.

Summary and Implications: Twice daily oral penicillin prophylaxis was associated with an 84% reduction in the incidence of serious *S. pneumoniae* infection in young children with sickle cell anemia. Nearly one-quarter of children in the placebo group who developed *S. pneumoniae* septicemia died, all within hours of reaching medical attention. The preventive approach afforded by regular prophylactic penicillin is potentially life-saving in such rapidly progressive cases of pneumococcemia.

CLINICAL CASE: PROPHYLACTIC PENICILLIN IN SICKLE CELL ANEMIA

Case History:

A 2-month-old former full-term boy presents to the office for a well child visit. He is new to your clinic, having recently moved from another state. His birth history was uncomplicated, and he has had no medical problems. He takes no medications and has no known drug allergies. He is breast-feeding on demand and voiding regularly. He coos, smiles, and lifts his head when prone. His parents have no current concerns, but add that one test was abnormal on his newborn screen. They are not sure what the problem was because they had not had the chance to follow up with his prior pediatrician as planned.

On physical examination, the boy appears to be an appropriate size for his age. He is well-appearing and cooperative. His vital signs are normal, and the remainder of his exam is completely unremarkable.

As you begin to discuss the list of recommended vaccines, your medical assistant enters the room with an update. Faxed records from the prior pediatrician's office just arrived and revealed that the boy has screened positive for sickle cell anemia. What additional item should you add to today's plan to ensure his risk of pneumococcal infection is reduced?

Suggested Answer:

Given his positive screen for sickle cell anemia—by definition, this is hemoglobin SS disease—the best way to decrease his risk for severe pneumococcal illness is to prescribe penicillin V potassium 125 mg by mouth twice daily and administer pneumococcal vaccine. Further tests should be ordered to confirm the diagnosis. In the meantime, explain the typical course of sickle cell anemia to the family and emphasize the importance of consistently taking penicillin to decrease the chances of life-threatening infection. Make arrangements for specialist care, so that comprehensive health supervision may be established.

References

1. Gaston et al. Prophylaxis with oral penicillin in children with sickle cell anemia. *N Engl J Med.* 1986;314:1593–1599.
2. Hirst C et al. Prophylactic antibiotics for preventing pneumococcal infection in children with sickle cell disease. *Cochrane Database Syst Rev.* 2014;(11):CD003427.
3. Falletta JM et al. Discontinuing penicillin prophylaxis in children with sickle cell anemia. *J Pediatr.* 1995;127:685–690.
4. Yawn BP et al. Management of sickle cell disease: Summary of the 2014 evidence-based report by expert panel members. *JAMA.* 2014;312(10):1033–1048.
5. Adams R et al. Prevention of a first stroke by transfusion in children with abnormal results of transcranial Doppler ultrasonography. *N Engl J Med.* 1998;339:5–11.
6. Lee MT et al. Stroke prevention trial in sickle cell anemia (STOP): Extended follow-up and final results. *Blood.* 2006;108(3):847–852.
7. Ferster A et al. Five years experience with hydroxyurea in children and young adults with sickle cell disease. *Blood.* 2001;97:3628–3632.
8. Wang WC et al. A multicenter randomised controlled trial of hydroxyurea (hydroxycarbamide) in very young children with sickle cell anaemia. *Lancet.* 2011;377(9778):1663–1672.

Infectious Disease

20

Empiric Antimicrobial Therapy for Skin and Soft-Tissue Infections

MICHAEL LEVY

> ... *empiric* [community-acquired methicillin-resistant staphylococcus aureus] *coverage is not associated with improved outcomes in the outpatient management of nondrained noncultured* [skin and soft-tissue infections].
> —ELLIOTT ET AL.[1]

Research Question: Do outpatients treated empirically for nondrained, non-cultured skin and soft-tissue infections (SSTIs) require community-acquired methicillin-resistant *Staphylococcus aureus* (CA-MRSA) coverage?

Funding: National Research Service Award, Agency for Healthcare Research and Quality Centers for Education and Research on Therapeutics.

Year Study Began: 2004

Year Published: 2009

Study Location: Five urban pediatric primary care centers affiliated with Children's Hospital of Philadelphia. In the region, >50% of positive cultures from SSTIs are CA-MRSA.

Who Was Studied: Patients 0–21 years of age who presented with a first documented SSTI. The included patients did not have a drainage procedure or wound culture, which suggests the infections were nonpurulent.

Who Was Excluded: Patients admitted to the hospital the day of presentation, those who received only topical antibiotics or more than one systemic antibiotic, and those treated with any antibiotic other than beta-lactams, clindamycin, or trimethoprim-sulfamethoxazole.

How Many Patients: 584

Study Overview: See Figure 20.1 for a summary of the study design.

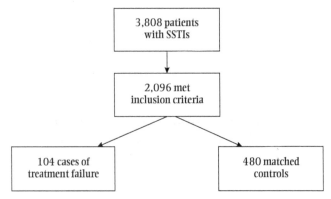

Figure 20.1 Summary of the Study Design.

Study Intervention: The initial course of antibiotic therapy was chosen by the treating clinician and consisted of monotherapy with a beta-lactam, which does not have CA-MRSA coverage, or with clindamycin or trimethoprim-sulfamethoxazole, both of which do.

Follow-Up: 28 days.

Endpoints: The primary outcome was treatment failure, defined as hospitalization for the SSTI or related complication, a drainage procedure, or a change or extension of the initial antibiotic course.

RESULTS

- Compared to those not receiving CA-MRSA therapy (beta-lactam therapy), those receiving CA-MRSA coverage with trimethoprim-sulfamethoxazole had a statistically significant higher failure rate (OR: 2.47 [95% CI: 1.41–4.31]) while those receiving CA-MRSA coverage with clindamycin did not (OR: 1.26 [95% CI: 0.71–2.23]).

- Other factors associated with treatment failure were fever at presentation, initial visit in the emergency department, and presence of induration or abscess.
- Of the included patients with treatment failure, an organism was isolated in 27.9%; 69% of those were CA-MRSA.
- During the study period, the proportion of prescriptions with CA-MRSA coverage increased from 16.4% in 2004 to 62.2% in 2007. The rate of treatment failure over this period did not change.

Criticisms and Limitations:

- While the data do not suggest that patients with SSTI who received CA-MRSA coverage had better outcomes than those not receiving CA-MRSA coverage, this was not a randomized trial and thus it is possible that unrecognized confounding factors may have influenced the results. For example, patients with more severe abscesses may have been more likely to receive CA-MRSA coverage, which may have resulted in similar or worse outcomes among this group.

Other Relevant Studies and Information:

- In a prospective study of adult inpatients with noncultured cellulitis, 73% were diagnosed with beta-hemolytic streptococci based on serology and blood cultures, and 96% responded favorably to beta-lactam antibiotics, suggesting a low incidence of CA-MRSA.[2]
- A randomized-controlled trial including patients of all ages showed no difference between cephalexin plus trimethoprim-sulfamethoxazole and cephalexin alone in treatment failure at 2 weeks and 1 month.[3]
- The 2014 guidelines by the Infectious Diseases Society of America (IDSA) recommend antimicrobial agents active against streptococci for mild and moderate nonpurulent SSTIs in immunocompetent patients. Clindamycin, which has coverage against CA-MRSA, is included as an option.[4]

Summary and Implications: Empiric therapy for CA-MRSA, versus standard beta-lactam antibiotic therapy without CA-MRSA coverage, did not improve outcomes, even in a region with prevalent CA-MRSA. Patients receiving trimethoprim-sulfamethoxazole, which has poor coverage for beta-hemolytic streptococci, had increased rates of treatment failure. This study suggests that CA-MRSA is not a major cause of nonpurulent SSTIs, and empiric therapy for this organism is not clearly warranted. For nonpurulent SSTI, guidelines recommend agents with coverage for beta-hemolytic streptococci as first line therapy.

CLINICAL CASE: EMPIRIC ANTIMICROBIAL THERAPY FOR CELLULITIS

Case History:
A 5-year-old boy presents to your urgent care clinic one evening with localized skin erythema consistent with cellulitis. There is no history of fever, no induration or spontaneous drainage at the site, and he has no drug allergies. What would you choose as initial empiric antimicrobial therapy?

Suggested Answer:
A beta-lactam such as cephalexin is an appropriate first-line choice. For cases of nonpurulent cellulitis, beta-hemolytic streptococci are the most likely causative organisms. Clindamycin would also be acceptable according to IDSA guidelines. If this child had risk factors such as fever or induration, stronger consideration could be given to CA-MRSA coverage. Trimethoprim-sulfamethoxazole should be avoided as it does not cover beta-hemolytic streptococci.

References
1. Elliott DJ, Zaoutis TE, Troxel AB, Loh A, Keren R. Empiric antimicrobial therapy for pediatric skin and soft-tissue infections in the era of methicillin-resistant *Staphylococcus aureus*. *Pediatrics*. 2009;123(6):e959–e966.
2. Jeng A, Beheshti M, Li J, Nathan R. The role of beta-hemolytic streptococci in causing diffuse, nonculturable cellulitis: a prospective investigation. *Medicine (Baltimore)*. 2010;89(4):217–226.
3. Pallin DJ, Binder WD, Allen MB, et al. Clinical trial: comparative effectiveness of cephalexin plus trimethoprim-sulfamethoxazole versus cephalexin alone for treatment of uncomplicated cellulitis: a randomized controlled trial. *Clin Infect Dis*. 2013;56(12):1754–1762.
4. Stevens DL, Bisno AL, Chambers HF, et al. Practice guidelines for the diagnosis and management of skin and soft tissue infections: 2014 update by the Infectious Diseases Society of America. *Clin Infect Dis*. 2014;59(2):e10–e52.

21

Infants at Low Risk for Serious Bacterial Infection

ASHAUNTA ANDERSON

We conclude that previously healthy infants younger than 3 months with an acute illness are unlikely to have serious bacterial infection if they have no findings consistent with ear, soft tissue, or skeletal infections and have normal white blood cell and band form counts and normal urine findings.
—DAGAN ET AL.[1]

Research Question: Can screening criteria be used to identify infants at low risk for serious bacterial infection?[1]

Funding: No external funding.

Year Study Began: 1982

Year Study Published: 1985

Study Location: Strong Memorial Hospital in Rochester, New York.

Who Was Studied: All infants younger than 3 months old hospitalized for suspected sepsis between July 1982 and June 1984 who were previously healthy defined as:

- Born full-term
- No perinatal complications
- No prior or current diseases
- No antibiotic treatment prior to evaluation

Who Was Excluded: Infants who were not previously healthy as defined above.

How Many Patients: 233

Study Overview: See Figure 21.1 for a summary of the study design.

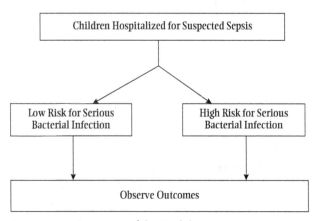

Figure 21.1 Summary of the Study's Design.

Management: All infants received the standard sepsis evaluation: complete blood count with differential; urinalysis; blood, urine, and cerebrospinal fluid culture; and cerebrospinal fluid cell count, protein, and glucose concentrations. Viral cultures were obtained within 24 hours of admission. It was also standard policy to administer intravenous antibiotics pending culture results.

Low Risk Criteria ("The Rochester Criteria"):

- No signs of ear, soft tissue, or bone infection
- 5,000–15,000 white blood cells/mm^3
- <1,500 bands/mm^3
- Normal urinalysis (≤10 white blood cells/high-power field in spun urine and no bacteria seen)

Outcome: Serious bacterial infection: bacteremia, meningitis, cellulitis, osteomyelitis, gastroenteritis, or urinary tract infection (>100,000 colonies of a single organism/mL)

RESULTS

- Infants categorized as "low risk" by the criteria were much less likely to have serious bacterial infections than those classified as "high risk," and none of the infants classified as "low risk" had bacteremia (see Table 21.1).
- Eight of the 9 high-risk infants with bacteremia had abnormal white blood cell or band counts.
- Low-risk infants were more likely than high-risk infants to have positive viral cultures ($P < 0.0005$).
- Age, sex, temperature, irritability, lethargy, anorexia, diarrhea, vomiting, respiratory findings, positive chest x-ray, cerebrospinal fluid pleocytosis, and isolated white blood cell count or band count were *not* predictors of serious bacterial infection.

Table 21.1. SUMMARY OF THE STUDY'S KEY FINDINGS

Outcome	Low-Risk Infants[a] (n = 144)	High-Risk Infants (n = 89)	P Value
Serious bacterial infection[b]	0.7%	25%	<0.0001
Bacteremia	0%	10%	<0.0005
Positive viral culture[c]	70%	41%	<0.0005

[a]Defined as no signs of ear, soft tissue, or bone infection; 5,000–15,000 white blood cells/mm^3; <1,500 bands/mm^3; and a normal urinalysis.
[b]Defined as bacteremia, meningitis, cellulitis, osteomyelitis, gastroenteritis, or urinary tract infection.
[c]Throat, stool or rectal, CSF, and blood cultured for viruses from July to November and nasopharyngeal or throat, stool or rectal, and CSF cultured for viruses from November to June. Respiratory syncytial virus and influenza A viral cultures obtained from nasal wash samples from December to May. Rotavirus cultured on per patient basis.

Criticisms and Limitations: In this prospective study, the authors did not perform the initial selection of patients with suspected sepsis. The pool of risk-stratified infants was established by the decision of house officers to admit the patient for sepsis evaluation. This may introduce some bias in the first round of study participant selection. It also means the study does not address the question of when to hospitalize infants for suspected sepsis or serious bacterial infection.

Study physicians were not consulted on the management of hospitalized study patients. Although the general policy was to administer intravenous antibiotics to all infants admitted for suspected sepsis, 33 of 233 did not receive intravenous antibiotics; none of the 33 had a serious bacterial infection. Therefore, the authors remark that the reported findings do not address the necessity for systemic antibiotics among patients admitted for sepsis evaluation.

Other Relevant Studies and Information:

- 1986: In a retrospective chart review of 117 febrile patients younger than 3 months old who presented to the emergency department, 3 of 70 (4.3%) infants classified as low risk by the *original* Rochester criteria actually had a serious bacterial infection.[2]
  - This produced a negative predictive value of 95.7% in contrast to 99.3% that was observed by Dagan and colleagues.
  - The false negative rate of 4.3% was considered unacceptably high given the low background prevalence of serious bacterial infection in this age group.
  - Because *Salmonella* infection was responsible for nearly all false negatives, the study authors suggested stool studies be added to the low-risk screen if other tests fail to identify *Salmonella*.
- 1988: In a study of 237 febrile infants younger than 2 months old, 148 were found to have a low risk for serious bacterial infection according to *modified* Rochester criteria that added 2 new stipulations: (1) <25 fecal white blood cells/high-power field in children with diarrhea and (2) no purulent otitis media.[3]
  - 42% of the low-risk infants were discharged home, 49% observed a short time and then discharged, and 11% were hospitalized.
  - No low-risk infants had a serious bacterial infection.
- 1994: Of 931 well-appearing febrile infants younger than 60 days, 437 met the once more *modified* Rochester criteria that now called for (1) ≤5 fecal white blood cells/high-power field in children with diarrhea and (2) no ear infection, purulent or otherwise.[4]
  - Five low-risk infants had serious bacterial infection, yielding a negative predictive value of 98.9% (95% confidence interval of 97.2–99.6%).
  - Study authors concluded the criteria were robust enough to consider observation of low-risk infants without antibiotics.

Summary and Implications: Febrile infants younger than 3 months with no history of medical problems; no evidence of soft tissue, skeletal, or ear infection; and who have normal white blood cell and band counts, and normal urinalyses, are at low risk for serious bacterial infection. The large majority of such infants will recover uneventfully.

CLINICAL CASE: INFANTS AT LOW RISK FOR SERIOUS BACTERIAL INFECTION

Case History:

A six-week-old former full-term boy is brought to the clinic by his mother with a history of tactile fever since the prior evening. He had an uneventful birth history, neonatal course, and has never taken any medications. He has been fussy with slightly lower oral intake since the onset of fever. His mother denies any other symptoms in the infant. She reports one normal wet diaper in the interim.

On exam, the boy is well-appearing with a rectal temperature measured at 38.2°C and mild tachycardia. All other vital signs are within normal limits. Assessment of the lungs, oropharynx, and tympanic membranes reveals no abnormalities. No tender joints or skin rashes are apparent. Capillary refill is normal and mucous membranes are moist.

Given the unremarkable exam, screening laboratory tests are conducted, revealing a white blood cell count of 16,000 cells/mm^3, 160 bands/mm^3, and normal urinalysis.

Based on the results of this study, how does this boy's risk for serious bacterial infection influence your management decision?

Suggested Answer:

It is appropriate to apply the screening criteria described in the study because this patient is younger than 3 months old, has no significant past medical history, and has not taken antibiotics recently. At six weeks old he is beyond the first month of life, which routinely indicates inpatient management with antibiotic therapy. He is also too young to avoid some portion of a sepsis evaluation.

He meets each of the Rochester low-risk criteria except the criterion for white blood cell count 5,000–15,000 white blood cells/mm^3. With 16,000 white blood cells/mm^3, he has a borderline placement in the high-risk category. While the tachycardia may resolve with treatment of his fever, his elevated white blood cell count and decreased oral intake may represent the first signs of a serious bacterial infection. He should be admitted to the hospital for further evaluation and treatment.

However, given his stable presentation and borderline high-risk classification, outpatient management with or without antibiotics could also be considered. These alternatives will be discussed in Chapter 22, "Outpatient Treatment of Febrile Infants at Low Risk for Serious Bacterial Infection," and Chapter 23, "Outpatient Treatment of Selected Febrile Infants Without Antibiotics."

References

1. Dagan R et al. Identification of infants unlikely to have serious bacterial infection although hospitalized for suspected sepsis. *J Pediatr.* 1985;107:855–860.
2. Anbar RD et al. Difficulties in universal application of criteria identifying infants at low risk for serious bacterial infection. *J Pediatr.* 1986;104:483–485.
3. Dagan R et al. Ambulatory care of febrile infants younger than 2 months of age classified as being at low risk for having serious bacterial infections. *J Pediatr.* 1988;112:355–360.
4. Jaskiewicz JA et al. Febrile infants at low risk for serious bacterial infection—An appraisal of the Rochester criteria and implications for management. *Pediatrics.* 1994;94:390–396.

22

Outpatient Treatment of Febrile Infants at Low Risk for Serious Bacterial Infection

ASHAUNTA ANDERSON

> *After a full evaluation for sepsis, outpatient treatment of febrile infants with intramuscular administration of ceftriaxone pending culture results and adherence to a strict follow-up protocol is a successful alternative to hospital admission.*
>
> —BASKIN ET AL.[1]

Research Question: Is outpatient treatment safe and effective for febrile infants 1 to 3 months old?[1]

Funding: Roche Laboratories provided ceftriaxone.

Year Study Began: 1987

Year Study Published: 1992

Study Location: Children's Hospital of Boston emergency department.

Who Was Studied: Well-appearing infants 28 to 89 days old with a rectal temperature $\geq 38°C$ who presented to the emergency department from February 1987 to April 1990 and met all of the low-risk criteria noted below.

Low Risk Criteria ("The Boston Criteria"):

- No signs of ear, soft tissue, or bone infection
- <20,000 white blood cells/mm³ (20 × 10⁹ white blood cells/L)
- Normal urinalysis (<10 white blood cells/high-power field) or urine dipstick test negative for leukocyte esterase
- Cerebrospinal fluid leukocyte count <10 cells/mm³ (10 × 10⁶ cells/L)
- No infiltrate on chest x-ray, if obtained
- No reason for hospital admission other than delivery of intravenous antibiotics
  - Normal vital signs for age and temperature
  - Not ill-appearing
  - Not dehydrated
  - Taking fluids
  - Reliable caregivers
- Caregiver available by telephone
- No antibiotics received in the preceding 48 hours
- No allergies to β-lactam antibiotics
- No diphtheria and tetanus toxoids and pertussis vaccine received in the preceding 48 hours

Who Was Excluded: Infants who did not meet the inclusion criteria described above.

How Many Patients: 503

Study Overview: See Figure 22.1 for a summary of the study design.

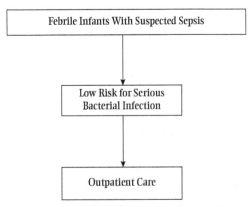

Figure 22.1 Summary of the Study's Design.

Study Intervention: Each subject underwent a complete blood cell count; urinalysis; cerebrospinal fluid analysis; and blood, urine, and cerebrospinal fluid cultures. An attending physician assigned each infant an Acute Illness Observation Scale score[2] (see Table 22.1). Chest x-rays and stool cultures were obtained at physician discretion. Infants who met the low-risk criteria received 50 mg/kg intramuscular ceftriaxone and were discharged home. They were reevaluated by telephone 12 hours later, in the emergency department with a repeat dose of ceftriaxone 24 hours later, and by telephone 48 hours and 7 days after study entry. Patients with positive cultures were immediately contacted and returned to the hospital for appropriate therapy.

Table 22.1. ACUTE ILLNESS OBSERVATION SCALE

Observed Item	Normal (1 point)	Moderate Impairment (3 points)	Severe Impairment (5 points)
Quality of cry	Strong with normal tone OR Content & not crying	Whimpering or sobbing	Weak OR moaning OR high-pitched
Reaction to parent stimulation	Cries briefly then stops OR Content & not crying	Cries off & on	Continual cry OR Hardly responds
State variation	If awake, stays awake OR if asleep & stimulated, wakes quickly	Eyes close briefly, awake OR Awakes with prolonged stimulation	Falls to sleep OR Will not arouse
Color	Pink	Pale extremities OR Acrocyanosis	Pale OR Cyanotic OR Mottled OR Ashen
Hydration	Skin, eyes normal AND Mucous membranes moist	Skin, eyes normal AND Mouth slightly dry	Skin doughy OR Tented AND Dry mucous membranes AND/OR Sunken eyes
Response to social overtures	Smiles OR Alerts (≤ 2 mo[b])	Brief smile OR Alerts briefly (≤ 2 mo)	No smile, Face anxious, dull, expressionless OR No alerting (≤ 2 mo)

Points for individual items are summed for total Infant Observation Score.
mo = Months old.

Follow-Up: 7 days. Charts of admitted patients were reviewed 3 to 12 months after enrollment. One of 503 patients was lost to follow-up.

Outcome: The primary outcome was a serious bacterial infection defined as: bacterial growth in blood, urine (>1,000 colonies of single organism/ mL for suprapubic aspiration sample or ^{3}10,000 colonies of single organism/mL for bladder catheterization sample), cerebrospinal fluid, or stool culture.

RESULTS

- Twenty-seven of 503 (5.4%) enrolled infants meeting low-risk criteria had a serious bacterial infection: 9 (1.8%) had bacteremia (including 1 with osteomyelitis diagnosed at 7-day follow up and 1 with a urinary tract infection), 8 (1.6%) had urinary tract infection without bacteremia, and 10 (2.0%) had bacterial gastroenteritis without bacteremia. All were well-appearing when recalled to the emergency department.
- Twenty-five of 27 infants with serious bacterial infection had stool guaiac or Gram's stain evaluated, which are not components of the Boston criteria. Of those 25 infants, 13 were identified as high risk by the modified Rochester criteria, another set of criteria described in other chapters of this book (sensitivity = 0.52).
- Of the 476 infants who did not have a serious bacterial infection, 453 (95.2%) were not admitted to the hospital and 23 (4.8%) were admitted for other reasons—including delayed ill appearance (2/476 [0.4%]) and parental concerns.
- Temperature, percentage of band forms, and absolute band forms differed significantly between patients with and without serious bacterial infection, but were not clinically significant due to small intergroup differences and large standard deviations (see Table 22.2).
- Age, Acute Illness Observation Scale score, white blood cell count, and percentage of polymorphonuclear leukocytes did not differ significantly between patients with and without serious bacterial infection.

Table 22.2. SUMMARY OF THE STUDY'S KEY FINDINGS

Characteristics	Infants with a Source of Bacterial Infection[a] (n = 27)	Infants without a Source of Bacterial Infection[a] (n = 476)	P Value
Age (days)	55 ± 17	54 ± 17	Nonsignificant[b]
Temperature (C)	39.0° ± 0.6°	38.7° ± 0.6°	0.01
Acute Illness Observation Scale Score (6–30)	8.0 ± 3.2	7.3 ± 2.2	Nonsignificant[b]
Leukocytes (10^9 cells/L)	11.3 ± 3.4	10.4 ± 3.8	Nonsignificant[b]
Polymorphonuclear cells (%)	35 ± 15	31 ± 14	Nonsignificant[b]
Band forms (%)	7.7 ± 6.1	4.2 ± 4.9	0.001
Absolute band forms (10^9 cells/L)	0.84 ± 0.72	0.44 ± 0.58	0.001

[a]Mean ± standard deviation reported.
[b]P values not reported.

Criticisms and Limitations: While most of the patients were spared the potential iatrogenic complications of hospitalization, all 476 patients who did not have bacterial disease and were not admitted to the hospital received antibiotic treatment. No ceftriaxone-related complications were observed for any enrolled patient, but continued widespread use may potentiate antibiotic resistance. In addition, while some families may have found comfort recuperating at home, some had anxiety regarding home care (at least 2 were admitted on parental anxiety alone), and some may have been unable to return to the emergency department for the required follow-up visits. Even with follow-up rates greater than 99%, 1 of 503 patients missed all of the planned follow-up evaluations.

Other Relevant Studies and Information:

- Eighty-six febrile infants younger than 2 months old identified as low risk for serious bacterial infection by the modified Rochester criteria were treated as outpatients with intramuscular ceftriaxone.[3]
  - One of the 86 infants had bacteremia and 5 were hospitalized for other reasons with no serious complications.

- Administration of intramuscular ceftriaxone and outpatient management of low-risk febrile infants was demonstrated to be the most cost-effective strategy compared to others such as universal inpatient treatment and selective outpatient treatment without antibiotics.[4]
  - A sepsis evaluation based solely on clinical judgment was deemed least clinically effective and ranked near last in cost-effectiveness.
- The Milwaukee criteria (similar to the Boston low-risk criteria except white blood cell count <15,000 cells/mm³ was used) reported only 1 serious bacterial infection among its 143 febrile low-risk four-to-eight-week-old infants discharged home after intramuscular ceftriaxone.[5]
  - Study authors estimate savings over $460,000 due to avoided hospitalizations.
- A literature review and expert panel approach was used to develop guidelines for the management of young febrile infants without a source of infection.[6]
  - Laboratory evaluation, hospitalization, and intravenous antibiotics were recommended for neonates, high-risk 28- to 90-day-old infants, and ill-appearing febrile infants of any age.
  - Low-risk 28- to 90-day-old infants may be managed as outpatients if appropriate follow-up is maintained.

Summary and Implications: Outpatient treatment is safe and effective for one-to-three-month-old febrile infants as long as they have a low risk for serious bacterial infection, and their caregivers are available for close follow-up by phone and on site. Under these circumstances, many infants may be spared unnecessary hospital admissions.

CLINICAL CASE: OUTPATIENT TREATMENT OF FEBRILE INFANTS AT LOW RISK FOR SERIOUS BACTERIAL INFECTION

Case History:
A seven-week-old former full-term girl presents to the emergency department with a history of fever for the past 8 hours. She "feels hot" all over, had not slept well during the night, and breastfed for slightly shorter intervals than usual. Her mother denies any other symptoms and says she just changed one wet diaper. She reports no complications during pregnancy, delivery, or since

hospital discharge. The girl has had no vaccines since birth, takes no medications, and has no known drug allergies.

On exam, the girl is well-appearing with a rectal temperature of 38.2°C and normal vital signs save a slight tachycardia. She is crying throughout the physical exam, but auscultation of the heart, lungs, and abdomen appear normal. Her capillary refill is brisk and she is making tears. No source of infection is evident.

Because no source of infection was identified in this febrile young patient, the standard sepsis evaluation is initiated. Screening diagnostics yield a white blood cell count of 16,000 cells/mm³ (16×10^9 white blood cells/L), 160 bands/mm³ (0.16×10^9 cells/L), normal urinalysis, and normal cerebrospinal fluid analysis.

Based on the results of this study, how does this girl's risk for serious bacterial infection influence your management decision?

Suggested Answer:

The study's screening criteria may be used to assess the girl's risk of serious bacterial infection because the clinical scenario matches the correct age range (28–89 days old), definition of fever (≥38°C), and nontoxic appearance on physical exam. At seven weeks old, she, like the boy in Chapter 21, falls into a category of patients that previously had little rigorous evidence to guide management.

She meets the Boston low-risk criteria as she has less than 20,000 white blood cells/mm³ (her count of 16,000 white blood cells/mm³ makes her high risk by the Rochester criteria), a benign exam, reassuring history, and normal urine and cerebrospinal fluid studies. If caregivers are available by phone and can return to the hospital 24 hours later, she is not only low-risk for serious bacterial infection, but also a candidate for outpatient management.

The girl may be treated with 50 mg/kg intramuscular ceftriaxone, discharged home, and followed up by telephone 12 hours later. A repeat dose of ceftriaxone should be given at a return visit 24 hours after presentation. There should also be plans for follow-up telephone calls at 48 hours and 7 days post-presentation. It turns out that in the study, a low-risk patient with the same age, temperature, white blood cell count, and band cell count[7] was later found to have an *E. coli* bacteremia. However, repeat cultures were sterile at 24 hours, so the patient was adequately treated. The patient was recalled to the hospital for intravenous antibiotic therapy when the first culture turned positive and made a full recovery.

Unlike the patient in this case history, many low-risk patients in the study had a viral infection and did not benefit from empiric antibiotic coverage. Chapter 23 discusses the safety of observing febrile infants without antibiotics.

References

1. Baskin MN et al. Outpatient treatment of febrile infants 28 to 89 days of age with intramuscular administration of ceftriaxone. *J Pediatr.* 1992;120:22–27.
2. McCarthy PL et al. Observation scales to identify serious illness in febrile children. *Pediatrics.* 1982;70:802–809.
3. McCarthy CA et al. Outpatient management of selected infants younger than two months of age evaluated for possible sepsis. *Pediatr Infect Dis J.* 1992;11(4):257–265.
4. Lieu TA et al. Clinical and cost-effectiveness of outpatient strategies for management of febrile infants. *Pediatrics.* 1992;89(6 Pt 2):1135–1144.
5. Bonadio WA et al. Efficacy of a protocol to distinguish risk of serious bacterial infection in the outpatient evaluation of febrile young infants. *Clin Pediatr.* 1993;32(7):401–404.
6. Baraff LJ. Practice guideline for the management of infants and children 0 to 36 months of age with fever without source. *Ann Emerg Med.* 1993;22(7):1198–1210.
7. The band cell count is incorrect in the original published article, but reflects the true value in this vignette.

23

Outpatient Treatment of Selected Febrile Infants without Antibiotics

ASHAUNTA ANDERSON

With the use of strict screening criteria, a substantial number of febrile one-to-two-month-old infants can be cared for safely as outpatients and without antibiotics.

—BAKER ET AL.[1]

Research Question: Is outpatient treatment of one-to-two-month-old febrile infants without antibiotics safe and cost-effective?[1]

Funding: No external funding.

Year Study Began: 1987

Year Study Published: 1993

Study Location: Urban emergency department in Philadelphia, PA.

Who Was Studied: Infants 29–56 days old with rectal temperatures ≥38.2°C who presented to the emergency department from July 1987 to June 1992.

Who Was Excluded: Infants who did not meet the inclusion criteria described above.

How Many Patients: 747

Study Overview: See Figure 23.1 for a summary of the study design.

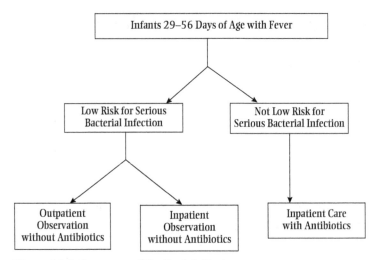

Figure 23.1 Summary of the Study's Design.

Low Risk Criteria ("The Philadelphia Criteria"):

- No physical signs or findings of bacterial infection
- Infant Observation Score ≤10
- <15,000 white blood cells/mm³
- <10 white blood cells/high-power field and few bacteria or no bacteria detected on bright-field microscopy of spun urine
- Cerebrospinal fluid leukocyte count <8 cells/mm³ in a nonbloody sample and negative Gram's stain
- No infiltrate on chest x-ray
- No obvious immunodeficiency syndrome*
- Band:neutrophil ratio normal (<0.2)*

*Part of the modified screening criteria added after the start of the study

Study intervention: History, physical exam, and Infant Observation Score were documented for each enrolled infant. After the standard full sepsis evaluation of complete blood cell count with differential; urinalysis with microscopy; chest x-ray; cerebrospinal fluid analysis; and blood, urine, and cerebrospinal fluid cultures, infants found to be not at low risk for serious bacterial infection were admitted to the hospital for antibiotic therapy. Patients with bloody cerebrospinal fluid specimens were also assigned to inpatient treatment with antibiotics. Stool culture and leukocyte analysis were obtained for those with a history of diarrhea. Those who met the low-risk criteria were assigned to one of two groups:

1. Outpatient observation without antibiotics if they presented on even-numbered days and if the following criteria were met:
   • Lived no more than 30 minutes away from the hospital
   • Had a working telephone at home
   • Parents were willing to return for reevaluation 24 and 48 hours later
2. Inpatient observation without antibiotics if they presented on odd-numbered days.

All infants under observation received inpatient care with antibiotics if symptoms worsened or cultures returned positive.

Follow-Up: 24, 48, and 72 hours for inpatients; 24 and 48 hours for outpatients; and 72 hours for cultures. No outpatients were lost to follow-up.

Outcomes:

• **Serious bacterial infection**: Bacterial growth of a known pathogen in blood, urine (>1,000 colonies of single organism/mL for bladder catheterization sample), cerebrospinal fluid, or stool culture; cellulitis; or abscess.
• **Serious illness**: Serious bacterial illness, pneumonia (new infiltrate on chest x-ray), or aseptic meningitis (≥ 8 leukocytes/mm^3 in nonbloody cerebrospinal fluid with negative culture an no recent history of antibiotic use).
• **Costs**: Length of hospital stay, intravenous therapy, and antibiotic treatment; complications; and total hospital charges.

RESULTS

The outcomes noted in Table 23.1 were observed for the enrolled infants.

- The Infant Observation Score did not reliably correlate with either the presence or absence of serious bacterial infection.
- If all 287 low-risk infants had been cared for in the outpatient setting without antibiotics, savings may have totaled more than $898,000.

Table 23.1. SUMMARY OF THE STUDY'S KEY FINDINGS

Disease	Inpatient-Antibiotic (n = 460)	Outpatient-Observation (n = 139)	Inpatient-Observation (n = 148)
Serious bacterial illness	64	0	1
Pneumonia	28	0	0
Aseptic meningitis	100	0	1
Otitis media	18	0	0
Viral illness*	250	139	146

Absolute number of infants reported.
*Viral illness includes diagnoses of viral syndrome, nonbacterial gastroenteritis, bronchiolitis, nonbacterial cystitis, and varicella infection.

Criticisms and Limitations: Under study protocol, a full sepsis evaluation is required with strict follow-up of outpatients to ensure safety. Smaller emergency departments may not be able to achieve the same level of patient outreach and follow-up. Similarly, some families may find it difficult to return to the emergency department for repeat evaluation. However, follow-up could be performed by the primary care provider as well. In addition, chest x-rays were performed for each infant, but only 28 of 747 were diagnosed with pneumonia. Thirty-four had bronchiolitis. Chest x-ray based on clinical indication alone may have significantly reduced the number of infants exposed to radiation. Of note, clinical indications other than fever identified only 23 of 28 infants with radiographic evidence of pneumonia.

Other Relevant Studies and Information:

- Study authors followed febrile infants 29–60 days old for an additional 3 years after the original 5-year study period ended, producing a total of 388 classified as low risk for serious bacterial infection.[2]

- None of the low-risk infants had a serious bacterial infection, resulting in a negative predictive value of 100% (95% confidence interval 99%–100%).
- Designation of febrile infants at low risk for serious bacterial infection produced similar results in a new cohort of 148 infants classified according to the Philadelphia criteria and 259 classified according to the Rochester criteria.[3]
  - Negative predictive value of the Philadelphia criteria was 97.1% (95% confidence interval 85.1%–99.8%) compared to 99.7% in the original cohort.
  - Negative predictive value of the Rochester criteria was 97.3% (95% confidence interval 90.5%–99.2%) compared to 98.9% in a prior analysis.[4]
- A literature review supported the use of low-risk criteria to identify febrile infants for management without antibiotics.[5]
  - The authors estimate that this strategy may help approximately 30% of febrile infants avoid complications associated with antibiotic use and hospitalization.

Summary and Implications: This study showed that febrile infants 1–2 months old may be safely cared for in the outpatient setting without antibiotics as long as a full sepsis evaluation—including both experienced clinical judgment and laboratory testing—and reliable follow-up are secured. It extends the work of Baskin and colleagues by demonstrating the efficacy and cost savings of outpatient treatment of febrile infants without antibiotics.

CLINICAL CASE: OUTPATIENT TREATMENT OF SELECTED FEBRILE INFANTS WITHOUT ANTIBIOTICS

Case History:

A nearly five-week-old former full-term boy is carried into the emergency department by his parents who report two days of worsening fever measured at 37.6°C orally just prior to presentation. He remains interested in feeding and has maintained his usual intake regimen. His parents have not noticed any change in his urine output and deny any symptoms other than fever. He has not been hospitalized since birth and has never been sick before.

On physical examination, his rectal temperature is 38.6°C and his vital signs are normal for the elevated temperature. He is cooperative and interactive with a normal Infant Observation Score. His skin is pink, and his mucous membranes are moist. There are no signs consistent with bacterial infection on examination of his ears, lungs, soft tissue, or bones.

Given his young age and normal exam findings, a full sepsis evaluation is performed. He has a white blood cell count of 14,300 cells/mm^3 with 1,000 bands/mm^3 and 10,000 neutrophils/mm^3. His urinalysis and cerebrospinal fluid studies are normal and nonbloody. Plain film of the chest reveals no infiltrate.

Based on the results of this study, how does this boy's risk for serious bacterial infection influence your management decision?

Suggested Answer:

As before, the first step is to ensure the screening criteria apply to this case. Similar to the infants enrolled in the study, this near-five-week-old fits the designated age range (29–56 days old), has a documented rectal temperature ≥38.2° C, and has no history consistent with immunodeficiency.

Despite his young age, he meets each of the Philadelphia low-risk criteria, both the initial set and the modified criteria, which add requirements for immunocompetence and band-to-neutrophil ratio <0.2. His white blood cell count of 14,300 cells/mm^3 is just inside the low-risk range. His band (1,000/mm^3) to neutrophil (10,000/mm^3) ratio at 0.1 is also in the low-risk range. According to this profile, he is a good candidate for observation without antibiotics.

In the study, low-risk patients were randomized to inpatient or outpatient observation without antibiotics. The study authors emphasize that both clinical and laboratory impressions must be considered together; neither is sufficient alone. Because this patient is near the newborn period with "worsening" fever per parental report, no clear source of infection after two days, and a borderline elevated white blood cell count, a conservative management strategy is in order. It is unclear why his parents waited two days to bring their febrile infant to medical attention, so there may be obstacles that prevent safe outpatient management. He should be admitted to the hospital where he can be closely monitored. The decision to begin antibiotics should be based on the subsequent clinical course. Observation without antibiotics is supported by the study and appropriate for this patient.

References

1. Baker MD et al. Outpatient management without antibiotics of fever in selected infants. *NEJM*. 1993;329(20):1237–1441.
2. Baker MD et al. The efficacy of routine outpatient management without antibiotics of fever in selected infants. *Pediatrics*. 1999;103:627–631.
3. Garra G et al. Reappraisal of criteria used to predict serious bacterial illness in febrile infants less than 8 weeks of age. *Acad Emerg Med*. 2005;12(10):921–925.
4. Jaskiewicz JA et al. Febrile infants at low risk for serious bacterial infection—An appraisal of the Rochester criteria and implications for management. *Pediatrics*. 1994;94:390–396.
5. Huppler AR et al. Performance of low-risk criteria in the evaluation of young infants with fever: Review of the literature. *Pediatrics*. 2010;125:228–233.

Neonatal Fever without a Source

ASHAUNTA ANDERSON

Unlike that for older 1- to 2-month-old [febrile infants] ... the Philadelphia protocol lacks the sensitivity and negative predictive value to identify neonates at low risk for [serious bacterial infection].

—BAKER ET AL.[1]

Research Questions: (1) Do infants in the first month of life (neonates) have the same profile of febrile illnesses as those in the second and third months of life? And (2) Can selected febrile neonates be safely and effectively managed as outpatients?[1]

Funding: No external funding.

Year Study Began: 1994

Year Study Published: 1996

Study Location: Children's Hospital of Philadelphia emergency department.

Who Was Studied: Infants 3–28 days old with rectal temperatures ≥38.0°C.

Who Was Excluded: Infants who did not meet the inclusion criteria specified above.

How Many Patients: 254

Study Overview: See Figure 24.1 for a summary of the study design.

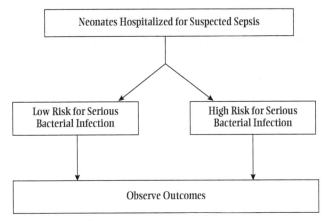

Figure 24.1 Summary of the Study's Design.

Low Risk Criteria ("The Modified Philadelphia Criteria"):

- Clinically appears well
- No signs of bacterial infection
- <15,000 white blood cells/mm³ (15×10^9/L)
- <10 white blood cells/high-power field and no bacteria detected on bright-field microscopy of spun urine
- Cerebrospinal fluid leukocyte count <8 cells/mm³ (8 cells/μL) in a non-bloody sample and negative Gram stain
- No infiltrate on chest x-ray
- Band-to-neutrophil ratio <0.2
- No blood detected in stool specimen

Study Intervention: History, physical exam, and clinical appearance were documented for each enrolled infant. Each infant received a complete blood cell count with differential; urinalysis with microscopy; chest x-ray, cerebrospinal fluid analysis; and blood, urine, and cerebrospinal fluid cultures. Stool bacterial culture, occult blood, and leukocyte count were obtained from those with a history of diarrhea. All infants were admitted to the hospital for intravenous antibiotic therapy. The modified Philadelphia low-risk criteria—which were initially formulated for one-to-two-month-old infants—were retrospectively applied to the enrolled cohort of neonates.

Follow-Up: 72 hours for inpatients and negative cultures.

Outcomes: The primary outcome was the presence of a serious bacterial infection defined as bacterial growth of a known pathogen in blood, urine (>1,000 colonies of single known urinary pathogen/mL for bladder catheterization sample), cerebrospinal fluid, or stool culture; cellulitis; or abscess. Pneumonia was considered a serious bacterial infection only if bacterial cultures of the blood or respiratory tract were positive for a known respiratory bacterial pathogen.

RESULTS

- Febrile neonates had a similar incidence of serious bacterial infections (12.6%; 32 of 254) as one-to-two-month-old febrile infants (10.2%; 43 of 422).
  - The 2 age groups also shared a similar distribution of bacterial diseases with urinary tract infections occurring more often than other bacterial diseases (see Table 24.1).
- Five of the 32 neonates diagnosed with serious bacterial infections met all of the low-risk criteria:
  - 2 with urinary tract infections
  - 2 with bacteremia
  - 1 with bacterial gastroenteritis
- The modified Philadelphia criteria have a negative predictive value of 95.4% (95% confidence interval 90%–99%), so of every 100 neonates classified as low risk, up to 10 neonates actually do have serious bacterial infection.
  - Positive predictive value was 18.6% (95% confidence interval 12%–25%)
  - Sensitivity was 84.4% (95% confidence interval 67%–95%)
  - Specificity was 46.8% (95% confidence interval 40%–53%)

Table 24.1. SUMMARY OF THE STUDY'S KEY FINDING

Classification	Neonates with SBI[a]	Neonates without SBI	Total
High risk for SBI	27	118	145
Low risk for SBI	5	104	109
Total	32	222	254

Absolute number of neonates reported.
[a]Serious bacterial infection.

Criticisms and Limitations: A major strength of the study is its ability to compare febrile illness in neonates to that in the older infants previously evaluated by the study authors.[2] However, only descriptive comparisons were made between the neonatal age group and the one-to-two-month-old age group, and the study was not powered to compare the incidence of final diagnoses between the two age groups. In addition, the similar overall rates of serious bacterial infection between the two groups were not compared statistically to confirm nonsignificance.

Other Relevant Studies and Information:

- In a study of 250 febrile neonates (28 days of age or less), those at low risk for serious bacterial infection were classified by the Rochester criteria with the additional requirement for a serum C-reactive protein < 20 mg/L[3].
  - Only 1 of the 131 low-risk neonates hospitalized without antibiotics had a serious bacterial infection (a urinary tract infection).
  - All inpatients required very close follow-up as 58 low-risk neonates were later reclassified as high-risk and started on antibiotics.
- The Rochester criteria were applied to a cohort of 134 neonates—this time the modified criteria calling for ≤5 white blood cells/high-power field in the stool specimen.[4]
  - Three of the 48 retrospectively identified low-risk neonates actually had a serious bacterial infection.
- Both the Boston and Philadelphia criteria were retrospectively applied to a cohort of 372 febrile neonates with similar performance: approximately 3% of newborns with a serious bacterial infection would have been discharged home (negative predictive value 97%).[5]
- A literature review and expert panel approach were used to develop guidelines for the management of young febrile infants without a source of infection.[6]
  - Standard full sepsis evaluation (blood, urine, and cerebrospinal fluid cultures; complete blood count with differential; urinalysis; and cerebrospinal fluid analysis for cells, glucose, and protein), hospitalization, and intravenous antibiotics are advised for neonates.

Summary and Implications: The modified Philadelphia criteria's low-risk classification included a number of high-risk neonates who were later diagnosed with serious bacterial disease. Although some studies have demonstrated the feasibility of inpatient management without antibiotics or outpatient management, current guidelines recommend that all febrile neonates be fully evaluated, treated, and remain hospitalized until bacterial culture results are known.

CLINICAL CASE: NEONATAL FEVER WITHOUT A SOURCE

Case History:

A two-week-old former full-term boy presents to his pediatrician's office for a health supervision visit. His mother is concerned he may be coming down with the same cold his two-year-old sister has. She measured his rectal temperature at 39°C this morning, but has not noted any other symptoms. He has been breastfeeding on demand, averaging about 1 feeding every 2 hours. He has had a wet diaper after nearly every feeding and several yellow, seedy stools per day.

Prior to the physical exam, he is sleeping in his mother's arms, but awakens easily and remains alert. He is nontoxic appearing and responds appropriately to stimuli. His rectal temperature is confirmed at 39°C with otherwise normal vital signs. Examination of the ears, oropharynx, chest, and abdomen are unrevealing. Capillary refill is less than 2 seconds. He has no rashes or tender joints.

Given the results of this study, how does this boy's risk for serious bacterial infection influence your management decision?

Suggested Answer:

Based on the observations of the study authors, this febrile newborn boy is likely to have a similar incidence of serious bacterial infection as older febrile infants. However, application of the modified Philadelphia criteria in his age group does not perform as well as in the one-to-two-month-old group. Moreover, other low-risk criteria have similarly failed to consistently identify neonates who can safely undergo less intensive management.

It is likely that this boy has a viral infection, as is the case among the majority of febrile infants, but serious bacterial infection cannot be ruled out at this point. The best course of action is to admit the boy to a suitable facility and treat him with intravenous antibiotics until blood, urine, and cerebrospinal fluid cultures are sterile after an acceptable time period, typically 48 hours.

References

1. Baker MD et al. Unpredictability of serious bacterial illness in febrile infants from birth to 1 month of age. *Arch Pediatr Adolesc Med.* 1999;153:508–511.
2. Baker MD et al. Outpatient management without antibiotics of fever in selected infants. *NEJM.* 1993;329(20):1237–1441.
3. Chiu C et al. Identification of febrile neonates unlikely to have bacterial infections. *Pediatr Infect Dis J.* 1997;16(1):59–63.
4. Ferrera PC et al. Neonatal fever: Utility of the Rochester criteria in determining low risk for serious bacterial infections. *Am J Emerg Med.* 1997;15:299–302.
5. Kadish HA et al. Applying outpatient protocols in febrile infants 1–28 days of age: Can the threshold be lowered? *Clin Pediatr.* 2000;39(2):81–88.
6. Baraff LJ. Practice guideline for the management of infants and children 0 to 36 months of age with fever without source. *Ann Emerg Med.* 1993;22(7):1198–1210.

Serious Bacterial Infections and Viral Infections in Febrile Infants

ASHAUNTA ANDERSON

> *Our data suggest that the use of viral diagnostic studies in combination with the Rochester criteria can substantially improve the ability of clinicians to stratify infants according to their risk of SBI [serious bacterial infection].*
> —BYINGTON ET AL.[1]

Research Question: Does presence or absence of viral infection help predict a febrile infant's risk for serious bacterial infection?[1]

Funding: National Center for Research Resources

Year Study Began: 1996

Year Study Published: 2004

Study Location: Primary Children's Medical Center in Salt Lake City, Utah

Who Was Studied: Infants 1–90 days old with temperature ≥38°C who were evaluated for sepsis. Each had been discharged from the hospital after birth.

Who Was Excluded: Any infant who received antibiotics within the 48 hours prior to presentation or who received a dose of the oral polio vaccine.

How Many Patients: 1,779

Study Overview: See Figure 25.1 for a summary of the study design.

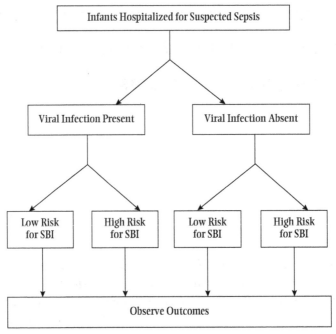

Figure 25.1 Summary of the Study's Design.

Low Risk Criteria ("The Rochester Criteria")[2,3]:

- No signs of ear, soft tissue, or bone infection
- 5,000–15,000 white blood cells/mm^3
- <1,500 bands/mm^3
- Normal urinalysis (≤10 white blood cells/high-power field in spun urine)

Study Intervention: Infants were enrolled from December 1996 to June 2002. Laboratory evaluation included bacterial cultures of the blood, urine, and cerebrospinal fluid. Other cultures and chest x-rays were performed for some infants with soft tissue infection, gastroenteritis, and pneumonia. In this sample, 1,385 infants had some form of viral studies performed:

- All enrollees were tested for enterovirus by PCR analysis of blood and cerebrospinal fluid or culture of cerebrospinal fluid, stool, nasopharyngeal, and throat specimens.
- Beginning in 1999, between November and April, nasal washes were obtained for detection of respiratory syncytial virus (RSV); influenza A and B; parainfluenza 1, 2, and 3; and adenovirus using enzyme-linked immunosorbent assay (ELISA), PCR analysis, or direct fluorescent assay detection.
- Rotavirus detection by ELISA and herpes virus testing by culture were performed at the discretion of the treating physician.

The Rochester criteria were applied to the portion of the sample with viral testing completed (1,385 of 1,779 enrolled infants).

Follow-Up: The exact length of follow-up was not specified.

Endpoints: The primary outcome was the presence of a serious bacterial infection defined as bacteremia, bacterial meningitis, urinary tract infection, soft tissue or skeletal infection, bacterial pneumonia, or bacterial enteritis. Secondary outcomes included physical exam data, diagnostic findings, antibiotic administration, and discharge diagnosis.

RESULTS

- Of the 1,385 febrile infants evaluated for sepsis and viral infection, 4.2% of those with a viral infection (21 of 491) had an SBI, and 12.3% of those without a viral infection (110 of 894) had an SBI ($P = 0.0001$) (see Table 25.1).
- One percent of those with a viral infection (5 of 491) had bacteremia, versus 2.7% of those without a viral infection (24 of 894; $P = 0.038$).
- Among the 922 designated as high risk by the Rochester criteria, 5.5% of those with viral infection had an SBI, whereas 16.7% of those without a viral infection had a SBI ($P < 0.0001$).
- No statistically significant difference in SBI rate was found between low-risk infants with a viral infection and low-risk infants without a viral infection ($P = 0.4$).

Table 25.1. SUMMARY OF THE TRIAL'S KEY FINDINGS

Rochester Classification	Viral Test Results	SBI[a,b]	Odds Ratio (95% CI[c])
Low Risk	Viral Infection Present	3/167 (1.8%)	1 (reference)
Low Risk	Viral Infection Absent	9/289 (3.1%)	1.76 (0.47–6.58)[d]
High Risk	Viral Infection Present	18/323 (5.5%)	3.23 (0.94–11.11)[d]
High Risk	Viral Infection Absent	100/599 (16.7%)	13.67 (4.27–43.72)

[a]Serious bacterial infection.
[b]Number of infants with serious bacterial infection/total number of infants in the risk-viral status subgroup.
[c]95% confidence interval.
[d]95% confidence interval that includes 1 indicates an odds of SBI that is not statistically significantly different from the reference.

Criticisms and Limitations: All enrolled infants did not have viral studies completed. In most of these instances, either parents did not consent to have the viral studies performed, or there was an insufficient sample for analysis. The incidence of serious bacterial infection in those without viral testing is not reported. Therefore, it is unknown if the group without viral testing was similar to the group with viral testing. This may bias the results in a direction that cannot be predicted.

In addition, the number of viral studies conducted varied from patient to patient. Viral infections may have been missed in patients with limited viral studies performed. Two important viruses, human herpesvirus 6 and rhinovirus, were not assessed in this study, which also may have led to the underestimation of viral infection in the sample.

Other Relevant Studies and Information:

- Among a sample of 1,169 febrile infants ≤60 days old, those with RSV infection had a lower risk of SBI than those without RSV infection (relative risk 0.6, 95% CI 0.3–0.9), but urinary tract infection remained significant in both groups (5.4% and 10.1% respectively).[4]
- For 809 febrile infants ≤60 days old, those with influenza infection had fewer cases of SBI than those without influenza infection (relative risk 0.19, 95% CI 0.06–0.59), but urinary tract infection once again remained significant in both groups (2.4% and 10.8% respectively).[5]
- A study of 1,125 hospitalized febrile infants 3 months old and younger found those with bronchiolitis had a lower incidence of SBI compared

to those without bronchiolitis (4% and 12.2% respectively, $P < 0.001$), but this was only true beyond the neonatal period.[6]

• After implementation of a care practice model based on the modified Rochester criteria and respiratory virus screening, 8,044 febrile infants experienced better outcomes and shorter hospital stays at reduced costs.[7]

Summary and Implications: Among febrile young infants with a high-risk Rochester classification, the presence of a viral infection is associated with a lower risk for serious bacterial infection. Rapid viral testing may facilitate early hospital discharge for appropriate high-risk infants with no viral infection. This is strengthened by the observation that the majority of bacterial organisms may be detected within 24 hours.

CLINICAL CASE: SERIOUS BACTERIAL INFECTIONS AND VIRAL INFECTIONS IN FEBRILE INFANTS

Case History:

We revisit the six-week-old former full-term boy discussed in Chapter 21 on serious bacterial infection. His mother reported less than 1 day of fever, some fussiness, and normal urine output despite mildly decreased oral intake. The boy had no other symptoms, no concerning past medical history, and no recent antibiotics.

He was well-appearing and interactive on physical examination. No signs of infection were appreciable. Because of his young age and febrile status, screening laboratory tests were performed, providing a white blood cell count of 16,000 cells/mm^3, 160 bands/mm^3, and normal urinalysis.

One additional piece of diagnostic information is now available. Rapid viral studies returned positive for respiratory syncytial virus.

Based on the results of this study, how does this boy's risk for serious bacterial infection influence your management decision?

Suggested Answer:

In the original discussion, it was deemed appropriate to apply the Rochester criteria because the boy was the correct age, younger than 3 months old, and previously healthy with no antibiotics on board. His classification was high-risk for SBI because his white blood cell count of 16,000 cells/mm^3 was outside the low-risk range of 5,000–15,000 white blood cells/mm^3. This laboratory value also classifies him as high risk by the Philadelphia criteria[8] (low risk requires < 15,000 white blood cells/mm^3). Therefore, a complete laboratory evaluation, hospitalization, and parenteral antimicrobial therapy were recommended.

There is now an important piece of new information. The boy is also positive for respiratory syncytial virus, which likely explains his febrile condition. It does not completely rule out the chance he also has a SBI, but, per the study findings, he is at lower risk for SBI than a similar high-risk child without a viral infection.

With a reassuring clinical picture, it would be appropriate to consider discharge after 24 hours of observation as suggested by Byington and colleagues. This entails obtaining at least blood and urine cultures. Cerebrospinal fluid culture is recommended if antibiotics will be administered. Discharge may be accomplished if bacterial cultures are negative at 24 hours, other standard discharge criteria are met, and reliable follow-up is planned.

Alternatively, if cerebrospinal fluid studies were conducted and normal for this infant at presentation, he would be considered low risk by the Boston criteria[9] (low risk requires < 20,000 white blood cells/mm^3) and eligible for outpatient management after intramuscular ceftriaxone. Of note, the Rochester, Philadelphia, and Boston criteria have been applied to the same patient for the purposes of instruction. Each provider and institution should select one approach to manage febrile infants and consistently apply it.

References

1. Byington et al. Serious bacterial infections in febrile infants 1 to 90 days old with and without viral infections. *Pediatrics.* 2004;113:1662–1666.
2. Dagan R et al. Identification of infants unlikely to have serious bacterial infection although hospitalized for suspected sepsis. *J Pediatr.* 1985;107:855–860.
3. Dagan R et al. Ambulatory care of febrile infants younger than 2 months of age classified as being at low risk for having serious bacterial infections. *J Pediatr.* 1988;112:355–360.
4. Levine DA et al. Risk of serious bacterial infection in young febrile infants with respiratory syncytial virus infections. *Pediatrics.* 2004;113:1728–1734.
5. Krief WI et al. Influenza virus infection and the risk of serious bacterial infections in young febrile infants. *Pediatrics.* 2009;124:30–39.
6. Yarden-Bilavsky H et al. Month-by-month age analysis of the risk of serious bacterial infections in febrile infants with bronchiolitis. *Clin Pediatr.* 2011;50(11):1052–1056.
7. Byington CL et al. Costs and infant outcomes after implementation of a care process model for febrile infants. *Pediatrics.* 2012;130:e16–e24.
8. Baker MD et al. Outpatient management without antibiotics of fever in selected infants. *NEJM.* 1993; 329(20):1237–1441.
9. Baskin MN et al. Outpatient treatment of febrile infants 28 to 89 days of age with intramuscular administration of ceftriaxone. *J Pediatr.* 1992; 120:22–27.

26

Chest Radiograph and Lower Respiratory Tract Infection

ASHAUNTA ANDERSON

The use of chest radiographs did not reduce time to recovery or subsequent health-facility use in children over 2 months with ambulatory acute lower-respiratory infection.

—SWINGLER ET AL.[1]

Research Question: What is the effect of chest radiography on the management and clinical outcome of acute lower-respiratory infections in ambulatory children?[1]

Funding: Medical Research Council of South Africa and the University of Cape Town.

Year Study Began: 1995

Year Study Published: 1998

Study Location: Outpatient department of the Red Cross Children's Hospital (Cape Town, South Africa).

Who Was Studied: Children 2–59 months of age who matched the World Health Organization case definition for pneumonia:

- Cough
- Tachypnea
  - ≥50 breaths/minute in 2- to 11-month-olds
  - ≥40 breaths/minute in children 12 months or older
- Drinking well
- No stridor, chest retractions, cyanosis, or mental status impairment

Who Was Excluded: Children with a cough for longer than 14 days, a current household contact with active tuberculosis, a focal wheeze, or clinical signs of heart failure were excluded. Children were also excluded when a clinician deemed chest radiograph a required part of the evaluation.

How Many Patients: 522

Study Overview: See Figure 26.1 for a summary of the trial's design.

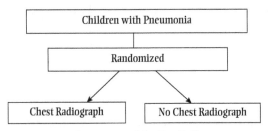

Figure 26.1 Summary of the Trial's Design.

Study Intervention: Chest radiograph (anteroposterior and lateral views) was performed for children assigned to the intervention group. Clinicians reviewed films and reports generated by the radiology department.

Follow-Up: The course of illness was assessed through twice weekly structured telephone interviews; only 295 of 522 could be contacted by phone. Any follow-up imaging, clinic visits, or hospitalizations were verified using medical records.

Endpoints: Primary outcome: Time to recovery (measured only in the 295 children whose caregivers could be reached by phone). Secondary outcomes: Tests ordered, number of drugs per prescription, antibiotic use, follow-up appointment, and immediate or later hospital admission (measured in all 522 participants).

RESULTS

- The median time to recovery was 7 days for both groups (95% confidence interval 6–8 days in the chest radiograph group and 6–9 days in the control group; $P = 0.5$ by log-rank test) (see Table 26.1).
- The hazard ratio for recovery in the radiograph group versus the control group (1.08; 95% confidence interval 0.85–1.34) was not changed when adjusted for age, weight for age, symptom duration prior to presentation, respiratory rate, clinician's pediatric qualifications, clinician's experience, and clinician's perception of need for chest radiograph.
- Children in the radiograph group were more likely to receive diagnoses of pneumonia or upper respiratory infection, while children in the control group were more likely to receive a diagnosis of bronchiolitis ($P = 0.03$ for comparisons involving each of the 3 diagnoses).

Table 26.1. SUMMARY OF THE TRIAL'S SECONDARY OUTCOMES

Outcome	Radiograph Group % (n)[a]	Control Group % (n)[a]	% Risk Reduction (95% CI)[b]
Initial Management			
Additional tests ordered	9.3 (257)	10 (261)	6 (57, –45)
Mean number of drugs per prescription	3.2 (245)	3.2 (255)	N/A
Antibiotic use	60.8 (245)	52.2 (255)	–17 (0, –33)
Follow-up appointments in 28 days	13.5 (245)	8.6 (255)	–56 (7, –120)
Hospital admission	4.7 (257)	2.3 (261)	–104 (25, –239)
Later outcomes within 28 days			
Follow-up visits to the hospital	32.8 (259)	32.3 (263)	–1.5 (23, –26)
Follow-up visits elsewhere	15 (139)	11.5 (156)	–31 (37, –99)
Hospital admissions	3.5 (259)	3.4 (263)	0 (91, –94)
Subsequent chest radiographs	7.7 (259)	9.1 (263)	15 (68, –37)

Table of findings adapted from Table 4 in the original article: Swingler et al. Randomised controlled trial of clinical outcome after chest radiograph in ambulatory acute lower-respiratory infection in children. *Lancet.* 1998;351:404–408.
[a]Percentage in each cell is followed by the number of children evaluated.
[b]Percent risk reduction is followed by the 95% confidence interval.

Criticisms and Limitations: A subset of the study sample could not be reached by telephone to assess the primary outcome, time to recovery. While baseline characteristics are similar for those with and without phone contacts, we cannot comment on time to recovery in the subset without phone contacts. Variables that influence phone access may also affect the value of chest radiograph for recovery.

The authors measure the loss-to-follow-up within the group with phone contact as 22%. Here, there are similar numbers of children lost from the radiograph group as the control group. Importantly, there is outcome concordance of the telephone records with the medical records reviewed for the entire group with phone contact (including those lost to follow-up).

Finally, some children were excluded because their symptoms were too severe, or clinicians felt a chest radiograph was required based on presentation. Therefore, this study does not apply to these children. However, medical record review of those excluded for mandatory chest radiograph did not reveal any benefit to chest radiograph.

Other Relevant Studies and Information:

- A 2013 Cochrane review[1] of randomized controlled trials on this topic reported no effect of chest radiographs on the clinical outcome of acute lower respiratory tract infection in children[2] and adults.[3]
- Guidelines produced by the Pediatric Infectious Diseases Society and the Infectious Diseases Society of America do not recommend routine chest radiograph for children with suspected community-acquired pneumonia who are well enough for outpatient treatment.[4]
  - They do recommend posteroanterior and lateral chest radiographs for children with hypoxemia, significant respiratory distress, or failure of initial antibiotic therapy.
- A prospective study of 507 children 1–16 years old with suspected pneumonia described the following predictors of focal infiltrates on chest radiograph[5]:
  - Fever
  - Tachypnea
  - Increased heart rate
  - Retractions
  - Grunting
  - Crackles
  - Decreased breath sounds

Summary and Implications: Chest radiograph did not reduce time to recovery for children 2 months old and older with ambulatory acute lower-respiratory tract infection. Further, no clinical subgroup of children or practitioner experience was found to modify the null effect.

CLINICAL CASE: CHEST RADIOGRAPH AND LOWER RESPIRATORY TRACT INFECTION

Case History:

A 6-year-old boy presents to the emergency department with a 4-day history of fever and cough. His mother states that he seems more tired lately and eats less, but has managed to drink plenty of liquids and maintain normal urine output. He has had some runny nose, but no trouble with breathing, vomiting, or diarrhea. His mother thinks he may have picked up the "bug" going around school.

On physical examination, the boy is alert and well-appearing with a temperature of 101.9°F, respiratory rate of 45, and oxygen saturation of 98%. He is breathing comfortably with no retractions or nasal flaring. There are mildly decreased breath sounds at the right anterior aspect of his chest. His mucous membranes are moist, and his skin is pink. Capillary refill time is less than 2 seconds.

Based on the results of this trial, should you order a chest radiograph to confirm the diagnosis of community-acquired pneumonia?

Suggested Answer:

This trial evaluated patients older than 2 months with mild pneumonia defined as cough and tachypnea without diminished oral intake, respiratory distress, cyanosis, or mental status changes. The boy in this vignette fits this description with his history of cough and elevated respiratory rate. On physical exam, his breathing is not labored, his skin is pink, and his mental status is normal. Of note, there are also no signs of focal wheeze or heart failure mentioned on exam.

The major finding of the trial was that chest radiograph did not speed recovery, so you should not order a chest radiograph for this boy. It exposes him to radiation without providing a health benefit. His mother may be counseled that he has pneumonia, and his symptoms should last a total of 7 days, plus or minus a few days. He should be discharged home on oral antibiotics.

This course of action is supported by the guidelines of the Pediatric Infectious Diseases Society and the Infectious Diseases Society of America, which are endorsed by the American Academy of Pediatrics. The guidelines also advise vigilance for failures of outpatient antibiotic therapy because this is an indication for chest radiograph. In this case, the imaging is needed to look for complications of pneumonia like empyema.

References

1. Swingler et al. Randomised controlled trial of clinical outcome after chest radiograph in ambulatory acute lower-respiratory infection in children. *Lancet.* 1998;351:404–408.
2. Cao et al. Chest radiographs for acute lower respiratory tract infections. *Cochrane Database Syst Rev.* 2013;12:CD009119. doi:10.1002/14651858.CD009119.pub2.
3. Busyhead et al. The effect of chest radiographs on the management and clinical course of patients with acute cough. *Medical Care.* 1983;21(7):661–673.
4. Bradley et al. Executive summary: The management of community-acquired pneumonia in infants and children older than 3 months of age: Clinical practice guidelines by the Pediatric Infectious Diseases Society and the Infectious Diseases Society of America. *Clin Infect Dis.* 2011;53(7):617–630.
5. Lynch et al. Can we predict which children with clinically suspected pneumonia will have the presence of focal infiltrates on chest radiographs? *Pediatrics.* 2004;113(3):e186–e189.

27

Vidarabine Therapy of Neonatal Herpes Simplex Virus Infection

JEREMIAH DAVIS

Superficial involvement of the skin, eye, or mouth, which appears to remain localized during the early course of infection, carries a far better prognosis than the other forms of neonatal herpes simplex virus infection.

—WHITLEY ET AL.[1]

Research Question: Does treatment of newborns infected with herpes simplex virus (HSV) with vidarabine reduce morbidity and mortality?[1]

Funding: The National Institute for Allergy and Infectious Disease (NIAID) contracts NO-1-AI-22532 and CA-13148, RR-032; Robert Meyer Foundation; vidarabine and placebo supplied by Warner-Lambert/Parke-Davis Research Division, Ann Arbor, MI.

Year Study Began: 1974

Year Study Published: 1980

Study Location: 15 hospitals throughout the United States.

Who Was Studied: Newborn infants presenting in the first month of life with confirmed HSV infection. Extent of HSV infection was categorized as

disseminated (hepatitis, pneumonitis, or disseminated intravascular coagulation ± CNS involvement), isolated CNS infection, or as localized (skin, eye,
mouth lesions).

Who Was Excluded: Infants who presented after 1 month old.

How Many Patients: 56

Study Overview: See Figure 27.1 for a summary of the trial's design.

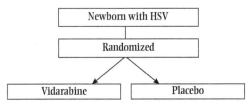

Figure 27.1 Summary of the Trial's Design.

Study Intervention: In a double-blind fashion, newborns with culture-proven
HSV infection were randomized into 2 groups: 28 patients received 10 days of
intravenous vidarabine and 28 patients received a placebo.

Follow-Up: Daily evaluations after enrollment until death or 30 days; then
assessments of neurologic status at 3, 6, 12, and 24 months after enrollment

Endpoints:

- Progression of disease—new lesions, neurologic signs, pneumonia,
  hepatitis, ocular involvement, associated complications or
  concomitant infection, or death.
- Neurologic or ocular sequelae, as well as recurrent skin lesions, noted
  at 3, 6, 12, and 24-month follow-up visits.
- Medication side effects.

RESULTS

- No significant difference existed between the study groups with
  regard to gender, race, gestation, birth weight, prematurity, disease
  duration prior to enrollment, or maternal factors.

- Of note, 7 of 63 originally enrolled patients were excluded from the efficacy analysis for higher than specified dose (2), a second course of vidarabine (1), or were given vidarabine for progressive disease (4).
- Mean gestational week for infected newborns was 36.4 ± 1.2 and 36.6 ± 0.8 for treated and placebo, respectively; duration of HSV disease prior to enrollment was 7.5 ± 1.2 days and 6.6 ± 0.9 days for babies in the vidarabine versus placebo, respectively.
- The mortality rate for both treatment groups combined was 70% for newborns with disseminated disease and 25% for those with localized CNS disease.
- For patients with disseminated and isolated CNS disease, vidarabine therapy significantly reduced mortality compared to placebo recipients at 6-month follow-up (74% vs. 38%, respectively, $P = 0.014$); 1-year mortality for all groups is listed in Table 27.1.
- Duration of disease, fever, cyanosis, and conjunctivitis significantly affected mortality rate; the improvement in mortality rates in the vidarabine group remained significant after adjustment for these factors.
- The sample size was too small to determine the impact of drug therapy on long-term morbidity. Compared to placebo recipients survivors of disseminated HSV infection did not appear to benefit from vidarabine; conversely, for localized CNS disease, 17% (1 of 6) of placebo patients were developmentally normal at one year versus 50% (5 of 10) of vidarabine recipients, suggesting some benefit on morbidity.

Table 27.1. SUMMARY OF THE TRIAL'S KEY FINDINGS (12 MONTHS)

Disease Type (Number of patients)	PERCENTAGE OF BABIES ALIVE AT 1 YEAR	
	Vidarabine	Placebo
Disseminated (27)	43%	15%
Localized CNS (16)	90%	50%
Combined—disseminated + CNS (43)	62%	26%
Localized skin, eye, or mouth (12)	100%	100%[a]

[a]A single patient in this group died during the study, but pathology revealed the cause of death was *S. aureus* septicemia and pneumonia.

Criticisms and Limitations: While this study was large enough to evaluate mortality, the sample size did not allow for evaluation of morbidity. The HSV status of mothers, presence of lesions at the time of birth, and method of delivery (vaginal vs. C-section) were not studied. Finally, "four placebo recipients [were] . . . given the drug because of progressive herpetic disease," although the reason for unblinding these subjects is unclear. Why these patients warranted a departure from the protocol, and whether they should have been included in subsequent analyses, is not discussed.

Other Relevant Studies and Information:

- The same group went on to compare these 56 infants with 39 additional infants treated in open fashion with two different doses of vidarabine (15 vs. 30 mg/kg/day × 10–14 days); the additional patients had a similar reduction in mortality rate (40% with combined disease). They also found that treated skin, eye, and mouth disease still carried a risk of neurologic progression (12%).[2]
- A multicenter, randomized, blinded trial comparing vidarabine to acyclovir (both 30 mg/kg/day × 10 days) found no difference in mortality between the two treatments and had similarly low side effect profiles.[3]
- A Cochrane Database review in 2009 included both analyses and was unable to make a recommendation for one treatment or the other.[4]
- The Red Book recommends treatment of neonatal HSV infection with acyclovir, largely for convenience of dosing, administration, and lower likelihood of systemic toxicity.[5]

Summary and Implications: Untreated neonatal HSV infection carries extremely high mortality and morbidity rates; this trial was the first high-quality study to demonstrate a clear benefit of antiviral therapy in survival for disseminated, localized CNS, and combined forms of the disease. While the study was not powered to assess the impact of antiviral therapy on morbidity, it provided important insight into early recognition and initiation of anti-HSV treatment in this vulnerable population. Current guidelines recommend treatment of neonatal HSV infections with acyclovir.

CLINICAL CASE: TREATMENT OF NEONATAL HSV

Case History:
An 8-day-old male presents to your outpatient clinic for a 1-week postpartum visit. You note a lethargic newborn with significant jaundice and tachypnea on your examination. Pre- and perinatal history are remarkable for a group B streptococcus–positive mother who received adequate treatment prior to vaginal delivery; the mother notes 1–2 small red bumps that were present in the days leading to delivery, but this was never discussed at the time of delivery. Screening labs demonstrate an elevated total bilirubin and a chest x-ray is concerning for pneumonitis.

Based on the context this study provides, what management is warranted?

Suggested Answer:
Whitley et al. provided a sober description of the very high mortality and morbidity rates associated with neonatal HSV infection. The presence of hyperbilirubinemia and pneumonitis in this infant strongly suggests disseminated HSV, which carries the worst prognosis. Whenever HSV is suspected, newborns must be admitted emergently and undergo skin, eye, and mucous membrane swabs, as well as blood and CSF nucleic acid testing for the presence of HSV. Intravenous and topical antiviral therapy should be started as soon as possible; while this study demonstrated the benefit of vidarabine on HSV-infected newborns, guidelines now recommend acyclovir as the first-line agent due to convenience and lower risk for toxicity.

References

1. Whitley RJ et al. Vidarabine therapy of neonatal herpes simplex virus infection. *Pediatrics*. 1980;66(4):495–501.
2. Whitley RJ et al. Neonatal herpes simplex virus infection: Follow-up evaluation of vidarabine therapy. *Pediatrics*. 1983;72(6):778–785.
3. Whitley RJ et al. A controlled trial comparing vidarabine with acyclovir in neonatal herpes simplex virus infection. *N Eng J Med* 1991;324(7):444–449.
4. Jones CA, Walker KS, Badawi N. Antiviral agents for treatment of herpes simplex virus infection in neonates. *Cochrane Database Syst Rev*. 2009;(3):CD004206. doi:10.1002/14651858.CD004206.pub2.
5. American Academy of Pediatrics. Herpes simplex. In: Pickering LK, ed. *Red Book: 2012 Report of the Committee on Infectious Diseases*. 29th ed. Elk Grove Village, IL: American Academy of Pediatrics, 2012;398.

28

Early Reversal of Pediatric and Neonatal Septic Shock

MICHAEL LEVY

Early shock reversal and resuscitation consistent with the new ACCM-PALS guidelines by community physicians can be associated with improved outcome.

—HAN ET AL.[1]

Research Question: Do resuscitation consistent with American College of Critical Care Medicine–Pediatric Advanced Life Support (ACCM-PALS) guidelines[2] and early reversal of shock improve outcomes for pediatric patients with septic shock?

Funding: Emergency Medical Services for Children, Maternal and Child Health Bureau Grant; Laerdal Foundation for Acute Medicine; National Institutes of Health.

Year Study Began: 1993

Year Published: 2003

Study Location: Local community hospitals in the Pittsburgh area as well as Children's Hospital of Pittsburgh (CHP), a tertiary care facility in the area.

Who Was Studied: Infants and children who had presented to community hospitals with septic shock and required transfer to CHP for tertiary level care. Septic shock was defined as:

- Suspected infection on the basis of fever or hypothermia, and
- "Signs of decreased perfusion, including decreased mental status, prolonged capillary refill time, diminished peripheral pulses, or mottled extremities."

Who Was Excluded: Premature infants <36 weeks corrected gestational age.

How Many Patients: 91

Study Overview: This was a retrospective review of CHP's interfacility transport records (see Figure 28.1).

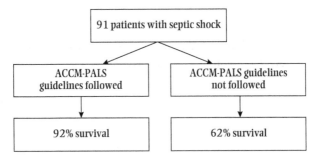

Figure 28.1 Summary of the Study's Design.

Study Intervention: Early resuscitation by community physicians consistent with ACCM-PALS guidelines. These guidelines include early recognition of decreased perfusion, and isotonic fluid up to and over 60 cc/kg in the first hour. If shock is fluid refractory, central venous access should be established and vasopressor therapy initiated.

Follow-Up: Patients were followed to hospital discharge.

Endpoints: The major endpoints measured were:

- Shock reversal (normal systolic blood pressure and capillary refill time)
- Hospital mortality

The authors recorded the frequency of 9 specific ACCM-PALS interventions looking for statistically significant differences between patients who were successfully resuscitated by community physicians and those who weren't. Pediatric Risk for Mortality (PRISM) scores were used to adjust for severity of illness.

RESULTS

- Resuscitation by community physicians followed ACCM-PALS guidelines in 30% of patients. Patients whose resuscitation was consistent with ACCM-PALS guidelines resulted in 92% survival, while resuscitation not consistent with ACCM-PALS guidelines resulted in 62% survival (see Table 28.1).
- Community physicians successfully reversed shock prior to transfer to the tertiary care facility in 26% of patients. Successful shock reversal in the community was associated with 96% survival, while persistent shock at time of transfer to the tertiary care facility was associated with 63% survival.
- Each hour of persistent shock was associated with increased mortality.
- Age, presence of comorbidities, transport time, and culture-positive sepsis were similar between nonsurvivors and survivors. Nonsurvivors had higher PRISM scores than survivors.

Table 28.1. SURVIVAL AND MORTALITY ODDS RATIOS
(ADJUSTED FOR PRISM SCORE)

Variable	Survival Odds Ratio	Mortality Odds Ratio	95% Confidence Interval
Resuscitation consistent with ACCM-PALS Guidelines	6.81	—	1.26–36.80
Shock reversed	9.49	—	1.07–83.89
Delay resuscitation consistent with ACCM-PALS Guidelines (per 1-hour increment)	—	1.53	1.08–2.16
Duration of persistent shock (per 1-hour increment)	—	2.29	1.19–4.44

Among the ACCM-PALS interventions studied, IV fluid therapy was particularly noteworthy. Community physicians administered appropriate fluid therapy ($\geq$60 mL/kg) to only 25% of patients who had persistent shock, and median total IV fluid volumes were similar between patients who had persistent shock (20.0 mL/kg) and those whose shock was reversed (23.9 mL/kg).

Criticisms and Limitations: The study is limited by its retrospective nature and the fact that it was not a randomized trial. Additionally, shock reversal was defined by clinical rather than invasive hemodynamic measures, which may have introduced interobserver variability. Duration of shock was measured beginning at presentation to the community hospital, but it was not known when each child first became ill. Patients were not followed beyond hospital discharge so morbidity among survivors is not known. Finally, timing and choice of antibiotic therapy were not considered.

Other Relevant Studies and Information:

- This is the first pediatric study to demonstrate that early, goal-directed therapy in the community can improve outcomes in septic shock. Using a larger prospectively collected database, Carcillo et al.[4] later confirmed reduced mortality with early shock reversal and resuscitation consistent with guidelines. They also demonstrated improved functional morbidity using Pediatric Overall Performance Category scores.
- Prior to this work, Booy et al.[5] reported a decrease in mortality of children with meningococcal disease after opening a new PICU and educating providers in the community.
- There is one randomized trial of fluid therapy in children with septic shock. The FEAST trial[6] surprisingly demonstrated increased mortality after fluid bolus in children with febrile illness and shock in resource-poor settings. However, this study may not apply in resource-rich settings with a different diagnosis profile and widespread availability of invasive monitoring and vasopressor therapy.
- More recently, Paul et al.[7] implemented a quality improvement project to improve adherence to national guidelines in an emergency department. They were able to significantly increase adherence to many metrics including the administration of 60 mL/kg of IV fluid in the first 60 minutes. They also saw an increase in the number of septic shock cases between each death.

Summary and Implications: Early reversal of septic shock by community physicians prior to transfer to a tertiary care facility reduces mortality in children. This can be accomplished by following the ACCM-PALS guidelines for early goal-directed therapy.

CLINICAL CASE: A PEDIATRIC PATIENT WITH SEPTIC SHOCK

Case History:

A child is brought to your community hospital emergency department with a fever. His mother reports that he seems confused. On examination you note weak peripheral pulses and a capillary refill time of 4 seconds. What are your first steps in management?

Suggested Answer:

This child is in septic shock based on suspected infection with signs of decreased perfusion. You know that rapid reversal of shock greatly reduces morbidity and mortality, and conversely each hour of delay increases mortality.

Your first concern should be for A-B-Cs: airway, breathing, and circulation. You should consider endotracheal intubation and mechanical ventilation. To support circulation you must first establish venous access and adequately fluid-resuscitate. If one bolus of 20 mL/kg of normal saline does not restore perfusion, you should continue to bolus up to and over 60 mL/kg in the first hour, or until normal perfusion is restored. Do not give repeated fluid boluses if there are signs of fluid overload such as rales, cardiomegaly, or hepatomegaly. Only after giving sufficient fluid volume should you proceed to vasoactive medications.

While this child may ultimately require transfer to a tertiary care facility, early care in the community according to ACCM-PALS guidelines aimed at quickly reversing shock is likely to result in a better outcome.

References

1. Han YY, Carcillo JA, Dragotta MA, et al. Early reversal of pediatric-neonatal septic shock by community physicians is associated with improved outcome. *Pediatrics.* 2003;112(4):793–799.
2. Carcillo JA, Fields AI. Clinical practice parameters for hemodynamic support of pediatric and neonatal patients in septic shock. *Crit Care Med.* 2002;30(6):1365–1378.
3. Rivers E, Nguyen B, Havstad S, et al. Early goal-directed therapy in the treatment of severe sepsis and septic shock. *N Engl J Med.* 2001;345(19):1368–1377.
4. Carcillo JA, Kuch BA, Han YY, et al. Mortality and functional morbidity after use of PALS/APLS by community physicians. *Pediatrics.* 2009;124(2):500–508.

5. Booy R, Habibi P, Nadel S, et al. Reduction in case fatality rate from meningococcal disease associated with improved healthcare delivery. *Arch Dis Child.*
   2001;85(5):386–390.
6. Maitland K, Kiguli S, Opoka RO, et al. Mortality after fluid bolus in African children with severe infection. *N Engl J Med.* 2011;364(26):2483–2495.
7. Paul R, Melendez E, Stack A, Capraro A, Monuteaux M, Neuman MI. Improving
   Adherence to PALS Septic Shock Guidelines. *Pediatrics.* 2014;133(5):e1–e9.

29

Reduction of Vertical Transmission of Human Immunodeficiency Virus

JEREMIAH DAVIS

Our study indicates that substantial reduction in the rate of maternal-infant transmission of HIV is possible with minimal short-term toxicity to mother or child.

—CONNOR ET AL.[1]

Research Question: Does zidovudine reduce the transmission of HIV from mother to infant at birth?[1]

Funding: National Institute of Allergy and Infectious Diseases, the National Institute of Child Health and Human Development, National Institutes of Health; Burroughs Wellcome Company, US; Agence Nationale de Recherche sur le SIDA, France.

Year Study Began: 1991

Year Study Published: 1994

Study Location: 59 centers in the United States, France, and Puerto Rico

Who Was Studied: Pregnant women between 14–34 weeks of gestation who were infected with HIV; mothers were required to have CD4+ T cell counts above 200 cells/mm^3 and to not have received antiretroviral therapy currently. In addition, mothers were required to have normal laboratory values for hemoglobin, platelets, alanine aminotransferase, serum creatinine (or urinary creatinine clearance), and absolute neutrophil counts.

Who Was Excluded: Mothers with ultrasound findings of oligohydramnios in the second trimester, polyhydramnios in the third trimester without explanation, life-threatening fetal anomalies, or fetal anomalies that could contribute to higher zidovudine concentration or its metabolites in the fetus. Mothers with prior antiretroviral treatment during the pregnancy, or those who had received anti-HIV vaccines, immunotherapy, radiation therapy, or cytolytic chemotherapy were also excluded.

How Many Patients: 477 pregnant women enrolled, 409 births involving 415 live-born infants.

Study Overview: Randomized, double-blind, placebo-controlled, multicenter, clinical trial (Figure 29.1).

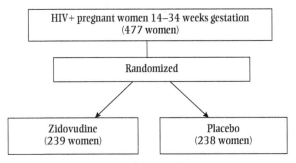

Figure 29.1 Summary of the Trial's Design.

Study Intervention: Women randomized to receive zidovudine were given antepartum zidovudine (100 mg by mouth 5 times daily) and intrapartum zidovudine (2 mg/kg IV for an hour, then 1 mg/kg every hour until delivery), and their infants were started on zidovudine orally at 8–12 hours of life (2 mg/kg by mouth every 6 hours) and continuing for the first 6 weeks of life.

Follow-Up: Postpartum women were evaluated at 6 weeks and again at 6 months after delivery. Infants were evaluated at birth, then again at 1, 2 or 3, 6, 12, 24, 36, 48, 60, 72, and 78 weeks of life. HIV cultures from infants' peripheral-blood mononuclear cells (PBMCs) were performed at 12 and 78 weeks of life; Western blots and enzyme immunoassays were conducted at 72 and 78 weeks of age.

Endpoints: Primary outcome: HIV infection of the infant, as determined by at least one positive HIV culture of PBMCs.

RESULTS

- Baseline characteristics of mothers were similar between both groups, including median gestational age of entry (and length of time of placebo or zidovudine treatment), CD4+ T cell counts, receipt of intrapartum infusions, and dose adjustments.
- Neonatal acquisition of HIV was determined by survival analysis (Kaplan-Meier) for the 363 births who had at least one HIV culture performed during the study period (180 infants received zidovudine, 183 received placebo); the estimated proportion of infected infants at 18 months of life was 8.3% in the zidovudine cohort (95% CI 3.9–12.8) and 25.5% in the placebo group (95% CI 18.4–32.5). This difference was significant ($P = 0.00006$).
- An alternate analysis defining HIV infection as 2 positive cultures and HIV negative as 2 negative cultures and no positive ones corroborated the previous analysis (Table 29.1).
- No adverse effects directly related to treatment were noted in mothers during the study period, and no maternal deaths occurred. CD4+ T cell counts increased significantly postpartum in both groups of mothers, but were higher among zidovudine recipients (though not significant compared to placebo).
- Infant or neonatal deaths occurred with the same frequency in both treated and placebo groups, and were not attributable to zidovudine. Post-neonatal deaths were due to HIV infection (2 zidovudine recipients and 4 placebo recipients) or to trauma (1 zidovudine recipient). Initial hemoglobin concentrations in zidovudine recipients were significantly lower, but by 12 weeks levels were similar to the placebo group.

Table 29.1. SUMMARY OF THE TRIAL'S KEY FINDINGS[a]

	Zidovudine	Placebo	P value
Infected infants >32 weeks of life	9 (7.4)	31 (24.4)	0.002
Total	150	149	
Infected infants ≥1 year of life	7 (8.4)	20 (22.5)	0.03
Total	95	104	

[a]Parentheses represent the transmission rate (%).

Criticisms and Limitations: Compliance with the intended treatment regimen was apparently monitored by self-report as no drug levels of zidovudine are reported. Similarly, HIV is transmitted by breast milk and breastfeeding was self-reported. A slightly higher number of women in the placebo arm did not complete their treatment (15 vs. 9) compared to the zidovudine group. Many of the intended subgroup analyses were not completed due to the small sample size of HIV infected infants in the zidovudine arm; a larger study size may have been able to adequately evaluate these subgroups.

Other Relevant Studies and Information:

- The same study group analyzed maternal blood samples from this cohort to identify any relationship between maternal HIV viral load and vertical transmission; they found that elevated maternal plasma concentrations of HIV was a risk factor for neonatal infection, but that reductions in viral load caused by zidovudine only partly accounted for the decreased transmission of the virus.[2]
- This study's findings were quickly adopted nationally and, in combination with routine HIV testing of pregnant mothers, the rate of vertical transmission in the United States dropped precipitously.[3] The advent of highly active antiretroviral therapy dramatically reduced viral loads in infected pregnant women, further reducing the incidence of neonatal HIV acquisition. A comprehensive look at the effectiveness of these interventions demonstrated that vertical transmission could be decreased from 22.6% to 1.2%.[4]
- Adoption of similar recommendations and national programs resulted in dramatically lower HIV infection rates in other countries as well, such as the United Kingdom and Ireland.[5] A large focus in the 21st century has been creating access to these simple interventions in developing parts of the globe, as affirmed by the US President's Emergency Plan for AIDS Relief in conjunction with the United Nations and World Health Organization.[6]

Summary and Implications: This trial demonstrated that maternal and infant treatment with an antiretroviral medication could effectively reduce the vertical transmission of HIV from mother to child. Such prophylaxis is now considered to be the standard of care. In the two decades since the trial, countries with access to antiretroviral therapy and comprehensive approaches to prenatal, perinatal, and postnatal care of infants at risk of vertical HIV transmission have seen dramatic decreases in infection rates.

CLINICAL CASE: PREVENTING HIV TRANSMISSION TO INFANTS

Case History:

You are rounding in the newborn nursery at your local hospital when the birthing center charge nurse pulls you aside. Overnight they admitted an HIV-positive mother at term who had rupture of membranes and is expected to deliver. She was on antiretrovirals prenatally with an undetectable viral load and is doing well. The mother is quite anxious about the risk of HIV infection in her infant and requested a pediatric consult to discuss the postpartum management of infants with known HIV-positive mothers.

Based on the results of this clinical trial and the guidelines that have been set out since its publication (http://aidsinfo.nih.gov/guidelines), what general treatment information can you share with the mother?

Suggested Answer:

After birth the infant should begin receiving oral zidovudine within 6–12 hours. This medication will be continued for the first 6 weeks of life. Typically a follow-up visit purely to check medication compliance is done at 2–4 weeks of age, and also to screen for zidovudine-associated anemia. An HIV DNA or RNA PCR is usually performed at 14–21 days of life; if negative, this is repeated at 1–2 months and a final time at 4–6 months. Of note, RNA PCR may be negative while the infant is on antiretrovirals; thus cell-associated HIV DNA PCR may be more helpful for diagnosis. If the infant is found to be HIV infected then an antiretroviral treatment regimen rather than zidovudine prophylaxis must be used. Also, it's important to educate the mother that HIV transmission can occur through breastfeeding, and that in developed nations it's advised that HIV-positive mothers avoid breastfeeding their infants to reduce the chance of infection. Many providers will confirm the HIV-negative status of the child between 12–18 months of age with a serum antibody test that should accurately reflect the child's circulating antibody levels, and not retained maternal antibodies.[7]

References

1. Conner EM, et al. (Pediatric AIDS Clinical Trials Group Protocol 076 Study Group) Reduction of maternal-infant transmission of human immunodeficiency virus by zidovudine. *N Eng J Med* 1994;331(18):1173–1180.
2. Sperling RS et al. Maternal viral load, zidovudine treatment, and the risk of transmission of human immunodeficiency virus type 1 from mother to infant. *N Eng J Med* 1996;335(26):1621–1629.

3. Centers for Disease Control and Prevention. Achievements in public health. Reduction in perinatal transmission of HIV infection—United States, 1985–2005. *MMWR*. 2006;55:592–597.
4. Cooper ER et al. Combination antiretroviral strategies for the treatment of pregnant HIV-1 infected women and prevention of perinatal HIV-1 transmission. *J Acquir Immune Defic Syndr* 2002;29:484–494.
5. Townsend CL et al. Low rates of mother-to-child transmission of HIV following effective pregnancy interventions in the United Kingdom and Ireland, 2000–2006. *AIDS* 2008;22(8):973-981.
6. Chi BH et al. Progress, challenges, and new opportunities for the prevention of mother-to-child transmission of HIV under the US President's Emergency Plan for AIDS Relief. *J Acquir Immune Defic Syndr* 2012;60(S3):S78–S87.
7. American Academy of Pediatrics. Human immunodeficiency virus infection. In: Pickering LK, Baker CJ, Kimberlin DW, Long SS, eds. *Red Book: 2009 Report of the Committee on Infectious Diseases*. 29th ed. Elk Grove Village, IL: American Academy of Pediatrics; 2012;418–439.

30

Palivizumab Prophylaxis against Respiratory Syncytial Virus in High-Risk Infants

JEREMIAH DAVIS

> *... palivizumab is safe and effective for prevention of serious RSV illness in premature infants (≤35 weeks gestation), including those with BPD.*
>   —THE IMPACT-RSV STUDY GROUP[1]

Research Question: Can palivizumab safely and effectively reduce hospitalization and other morbidity associated with respiratory syncytial virus (RSV) infection in high-risk infants?[1]

Funding: MedImmune, Inc.

Year Study Began: 1996

Year Study Published: 1998

Study Location: 119 centers in the United States, 9 centers in Canada, and 11 centers in the United Kingdom (139 total) participating in the Impact-RSV study group.

Who Was Studied: Children who met either of the following criteria:

- Born at 35 weeks gestation or younger and were ≤6 months of age

- ≤24 months of age with a diagnosis of bronchopulmonary dysplasia (BPD) defined as the use of diuretics, steroids, bronchodilators, or oxygen in the prior 6 months

Who Was Excluded: Children with active or recent RSV infection, those who had received a prior RSV immune globulin in the last 3 months or had ever received other experimental products (RSV vaccines, etc.), those with complicated or hemodynamically significant congenital heart disease, renal or hepatic disease, seizures, immunodeficiency, or who were currently hospitalized at the study's start with a length of stay anticipated >30 days or currently on mechanical ventilation.

How Many Patients: 1,502

Study Overview: See Figure 30.1 for a summary of the trial's design.

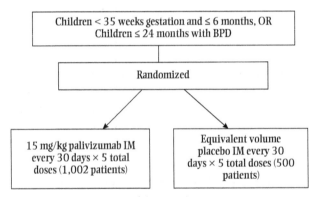

Figure 30.1 Summary of the Trial's Design.

Study Intervention: Children assigned to the study group received 15 mg/kg IM injections of a humanized monoclonal antibody against RSV (palivizumab) every 30 days for a total of 5 doses during the 1996–1997 RSV season; those assigned to the placebo group received an equivalent number of IM injections of a placebo.

Follow-Up: Children were followed until 30 days after the last scheduled injection (total of 150 days), with assessments at each injection visit and daily if hospitalized. Adverse events were monitored continuously during the study period; serum measurements were collected before the first injection and after the last injection of BUN, creatinine, ALT, AST, palivizumab concentration, and anti-palivizumab binding.

Endpoints: Primary outcome: hospitalization with RSV bronchiolitis confirmed by antigen testing of respiratory secretions. Secondary outcomes: incidence of otitis media, hospitalization for non-RSV-related respiratory tract disease, the total days of hospitalization with RSV, increased oxygen support, intensive care treatment, mechanical ventilation, and moderate or severe lower respiratory tract illness were followed.

RESULTS

- Baseline demographics between palivizumab and placebo groups were similar, with the exception of more palivizumab households containing at least one smoker in the household.
- Palivizumab prophylaxis resulted in a 55% decrease ($P = 0.0004$, 95% CI 38%, 72%) in RSV-associated hospitalization. Adjusting for BPD, entry weight, entry age, and gender this association remained statistically significant ($P < 0.001$) (see Table 30.1).
- Palivizumab recipients had significantly fewer total RSV hospitalization days, days requiring increased oxygen, and days with a moderate to severe lower respiratory tract infection; while fewer palivizumab recipients had ICU stays (and their stays were shorter), there was no difference in incidence or length of mechanical ventilation.
- There were no statistically significant differences in adverse events between the placebo and palivizumab groups.

Table 30.1. SUMMARY OF THE TRIAL'S KEY FINDINGS

Outcome	Placebo	Palivizumab	P Value
Incidence of RSV hospitalization—all	10.6%	4.8%	<0.001
Incidence of RSV hospitalization—premature (no BPD)	8.1%	1.8%	<0.001
Incidence of RSV hospitalization—BPD	12.8%	7.9%	0.038

Criticisms and Limitations: Hospitalization as the primary endpoint relies on individual practitioner decisions to admit, and admission criteria may differ between institutions. This may explain why a wide variation was seen in hospitalization reductions: 56% reduction in the United States versus 64% reduction in the United Kingdom versus 40% reduction in Canada. Uniform admission criteria could have strengthened the findings. In addition, the possibility of co-infections with other viruses or bacteria is not clearly addressed. Finally, patients with renal, hepatic, or significant cardiac comorbidities were excluded, as were those with seizure disorders or immunodeficiencies, and thus the results may not apply to these high-risk populations.

Other Relevant Studies and Information:

- This study was based on prior investigations that demonstrated RSV immune globulin could decrease serious RSV infections in high-risk infants[2,3] by passive immunization; unlike immune globulin, palivizumab does not require intravenous administration and does not carry the risk of bloodborne pathogen transmission.
- Palivizumab was widely recommended for high-risk infants following the Impact-RSV study, and two subsequent analyses of patients who received prophylaxis corroborated the low hospitalization rates for RSV among those who received palivizumab.[4,5]
- Since its release, overall rates of RSV hospitalization have declined, and preterm infants are generally healthier due to improvements in neonatal care; for these reasons, use of prophylaxis is now restricted to those infants born even more premature (before 29 weeks gestation) than originally studied, and for those with chronic medical conditions.[6]

Summary and Implications: Prophylaxis against RSV infection in high-risk infants (<6 months old and born prematurely ≤35 weeks gestational age) or children with BPD less than 2 years of age, results in lower RSV-related hospitalization rates, fewer days hospitalized, less need for supplemental oxygen, and

---

CLINICAL CASE: PREVENTING RSV IN HIGH-RISK INFANTS

Case History:

An 8-month-old ex-28-week premature female infant presents to your outpatient practice in December. The patient's neonatal course included 8 weeks in the NICU with a week of intubation, three weeks of noninvasive positive pressure ventilation, and required supplemental oxygen at the time of discharge. She had a grade II intraventricular hemorrhage but did not suffer any postnatal infections, hydrocephalus, or other long-term sequelae. She was able to come off home oxygen 2 months after discharge. Her growth and development are appropriate based on adjustment for gestational age at birth, and her parents ask about what they can do to help decrease her risk of "catching RSV"—which they learned about from an online forum with parents of premature infants.

Based on the results of this trial, what prophylaxis should you offer the family?

Suggested Answer:

In addition to discussing strategies to avoid infection (hand washing, avoiding known sick exposures) with the family, it is important to offer palivizumab prophylaxis for this infant. Her young age and history of prematurity qualify her as "high risk," and by administering the prophylactic antibodies prior to infection you can decrease the likelihood RSV-related hospitalization by over 50%.

less ICU care. History of prematurity should prompt practitioners to consider prophylaxis at the start of RSV season each winter.

References

1. The ImpactRSV Study Group. Palivizumab, a humanized respiratory syncytial virus monoclonal antibody, reduces hospitalization from respiratory syncytial virus infection in high-risk infants. *Pediatrics.* 1998;102(3):531–537.
2. Groothuis JR, Simoes EAF, Levin MJ, et al. Prophylactic administration of respiratory syncytial virus immune globulin to high-risk infants and young children. *N Eng J Med.* 1993;329:1524–1530.
3. The PREVENT Study Group. Reduction of respiratory syncytial virus hospitalization among premature infants and infants with bronchopulmonary dysplasia using respiratory syncytial virus immune globulin prophylaxis. *Pediatrics.* 1997;99:93–99.
4. Sorrentino M, Powers T. Effectiveness of palivizumab: evaluation of outcomes from the 1998 to 1999 respiratory virus season. The Palivizumab Outcomes Study Group. *Pediatr Infect Dis J.* 2000;19(11):1068–1071.
5. Lacaze-Masmonteil T, Roze JC, Fauroux B. Incidence of respiratory syncytial virus-related hospitalizations in high-risk children: follow-up of a national cohort of infants treated with palivizumab as RSV prophylaxis. *Pediatr Pulmonol.* 2002;34(3):181–188.
6. Committee on Infectious Diseases and Bronchiolitis Guidelines Committee. Updated guidance for palivizumab prophylaxis among infants and young children at increased risk of hospitalization for respiratory syncytial virus infection. *Pediatrics* 2014;134(2):415–420.

31

The Spectrum of Bronchiolitis

JEREMIAH DAVIS

The present study shows that if the clinician considers the age and sex of the patient, the season of the year, and has some knowledge of the characteristics of other illnesses occurring in the community, a remarkably accurate estimate can be made concerning the etiology of [wheezing associated respiratory infections].

—HENDERSON ET AL.[1]

Research Question: What are the characteristics of wheezing-associated respiratory illnesses in children in the outpatient setting?[1]

Funding: Vaccine Development Branch of the National Institute of Allergy and Infectious Diseases, NIH; US Army Medical Research and Development Command; National Heart, Lung, Blood Institute, NIH

Year Study Began: 1964

Year Study Published: 1979

Study Location: Single private pediatric practice in Chapel Hill, North Carolina.

Who Was Studied: Children 0–15 years of age seeking care for acute lower respiratory illnesses (LRIs) between 1964–1975. Symptoms of lower tract disease included wheezing (representing bronchiolar obstruction), retractions, and air trapping, with or without tachypnea. Lower tract disease was categorized as croup-laryngitis, tracheobronchitis, bronchiolitis, or pneumonia. Known allergic children were included if their wheezing occurred with other signs of respiratory tract infection.

Who Was Excluded: Children seeking care for other purposes at the pediatric practice or those over 15 years of age; children whose parents refused consent.

How Many Patients: 56,025 child-years were observed, with 6,165 LRIs studied; of these LRIs, 1,412 total patients were responsible for 1,851 wheezing-associated respiratory illnesses (WARIs).

Study Overview: Consenting children (per parents) were examined and had clinical and epidemiologic data collected, as well as throat culture for viruses and mycoplasma sent. Clinical, epidemiological, and laboratory results were recorded and data were analyzed for age, sex, etiologic, and epidemiologic characteristics of WARIs.

RESULTS

- During the study period 6,165 LRIs were studied, of which 1,851 (30% of all LRIs) had a significant component of wheezing (found in 1,412 different children).
- The highest incidence of WARIs occurred in the first year of life (11.4 cases per 100 children per year), falling sharply every year thereafter: 6.0 cases per 100 children per year from 12–24 months, and 1.3 cases per 100 children per year in elementary school.
- Males were more likely to experience WARIs until age 9 years, after which the risk was equal between genders.
- Of the 1,851 WARIs, 396 had nonbacterial respiratory pathogens isolated (21% of all WARIs); 87% of these were accounted for by respiratory syncytial virus (RSV), adenovirus (AV), rhinovirus (RV), parainfluenza virus (P1 and P3), and *Mycoplasma pneumoniae* (MP); these isolates demonstrated that RSV was the most common cause in preschool children, while *M. pneumoniae* was the most common at school age (Table 31.1).
- While wheezing was noted most commonly in LRIs from rhinovirus (49%), RSV (38%), and adenoviruses (35.9%), all isolates from LRIs had associations with wheezing.
- Seasonal associations between WARIs were noted, with winter months corresponding to increased isolates from LRIs; for 0–2 year olds RSV was associated with WARI epidemics; 2–5 year olds demonstrated correlation with RSV outbreaks, parainfluenzae, as well as *M. pneumoniae*; 5 years and older correlated with *M. pneumoniae* and to a lesser extent parainfluenzae outbreaks.

Table 31.1. SUMMARY OF THE TRIAL'S KEY FINDINGS

Age (Yr)	Cases of WARI	Total with Isolate	AGENTS[a]					
			RSV	P1	P3	AV	RV	MP
0–2	909	203	90 (44.3)	26 (12.8)	28 (13.8)	27 (13.3)	9 (4.4)	6 (3.0)
2–5	542	117	36 (30.8)	14 (12)	21 (17.9)	12 (10.3)	5 (4.3)	13 (11.1)
5–9	275	57	7 (12.3)	6 (10.5)	7 (12.3)	3 (5.3)	8 (14.0)	17 (29.8)
9–15	125	19	2 (10.5)	3 (15.8)	1 (5.3)	0	2 (10.5)	10 (52.6)
All ages	1,851	396	135 (34.1)	49 (12.4)	57 (14.4)	42 (10.6)	24 (6.1)	46 (11.6)

[a]Number of isolates; parentheses represent percent of total with isolates. RSV—respiratory syncytial virus; P1—parainfluenzae type 1; P3—parainfluenzae type 3; AV—adenoviruses; RV—rhinoviruses; MP—*M. pneumoniae.*

Criticisms and Limitations: This study was performed in a single center with a group of initially two pediatricians that grew to a total of four. The inclusion of patients depended on the clinical categorization of their illness as lower respiratory tract, which was not corroborated with imaging or any other modality. Additionally, there are no descriptions of interobserver variability or reliability between different practitioners' assessments. There is no report of how many parents declined participation, so it is unknown what fraction of the children studied represented all children presenting with LRIs to the practice. Throat swabs were used to determine etiologic agents of lower tract illness, but it is now known that the agents present in the oropharynx may not accurately describe lower respiratory tract pathogens. Similarly, newer methods of detection (such as polymerase chain reaction) have a much greater sensitivity, and if the same samples were analyzed using PCR, they might yield additional etiologic agents. Additionally, "croup-laryngitis" is discussed as a single entity, while currently these are managed as distinct clinical entities. Only a fifth of all WARIs had a positive agent identified, making the generalizability of these findings quite difficult.

Other Relevant Studies and Information:

- This group also published studies analyzing respiratory infections utilizing data from their outpatient private practice and a local university daycare[2]; they also studied the epidemiology and etiology of croup[3] and tracheobronchitis.[4] All of these findings were published in a comprehensive review.[5] The descriptions of the incidence and etiologic agents for these common outpatient diseases were some of the first reported from outpatient pediatric settings.
- Subsequent studies have further delineated the importance of RSV in bronchiolitis,[6,7] though human rhinovirus has increasingly been recognized as an important etiology of this disease.[8]

- The connection between LRIs and wheezing has also become an area of active investigation, particularly the relationship between childhood LRIs and the development of asthma. Findings from Tucson, Arizona have revealed that early childhood wheezing from LRIs may represent a different phenotype than childhood atopic asthmatics, and that these differences persist at least through adolescence.[9,10]

Summary and Implications: This study is a prospective cohort study that describes characteristics of wheezing associated respiratory illnesses in an outpatient setting. It showed that WARIs were common presentations of LRIs—even among older school-aged children, and that by utilizing age and season a reasonable guess could be made as to the most likely etiologic agents. They also helped confirm the principal role of RSV in WARIs in those <2 years of age, and in particular for infants. This finding helped direct future efforts at therapeutics and isolation strategies to curtail RSV infection in vulnerable infants and newborns.

CLINICAL CASE: WHEEZING IN OUTPATIENT LOWER RESPIRATORY TRACT INFECTIONS

Case History:

The parents of a 3-year-old male present to your outpatient office in October for low-grade temperatures, breathing fast, nasal congestion, and cough for the past 3 days. On examination you find a nontoxic child with rhinorrhea, occasional coughing, and coarse breath sounds bilaterally that have end-expiratory wheezes. His parents are concerned because he was hospitalized overnight at 4 months of age for bronchiolitis. They want to know if he's caught RSV again and whether he's likely to need inpatient treatment again.

Based on the findings of Henderson et al., what can you tell them?

Suggested Answer:

Henderson et al. found that wheezing associated with lower respiratory tract illness in outpatient clinics was more common in older children than previously described. While RSV is still an important contributor in children 2–5 years of age, parainfluenza, adenovirus, and *M. pneumoniae* were also seen in seasonal outbreaks to be associated with WARIs. Henderson and colleagues' data suggested that parainfluenza and *M. pneumoniae* were more likely to cause epidemics in October than RSV, and this hypothesis should be correlated with community lab data regarding current isolates. This patient's parents can be counseled that at his age, other agents are equally likely to be contributing to his LRI, and his clinical course will not automatically parallel the one he had as an infant.

References

1. Henderson FW et al. The etiologic and epidemiologic spectrum of bronchiolitis in pediatric practice. *J Pediatrics.* 1979;95(2):183–190.
2. Denny FW et al. The epidemiology of bronchiolitis. *Pediat Res.* 1977;11:234–236.
3. Denny FW et al. Croup: an 11-year study in a pediatric practice. *Pediatrics.* 1983;71(6):871–876.
4. Chapman RS et al. The epidemiology of tracheobronchitis in pediatric practice. *Am J of Epidemiology.* 1981;114(6):786–797.
5. Denny FW, Clyde WA Jr. Acute lower respiratory tract infections in nonhospitalized children. *The J of Pediatrics.* 1986;108(5):636–646.
6. Hall CB et al. The burden of respiratory syncytial virus infection in young children. *N Eng J Med.* 2009;360:588–598.
7. Koehoorn M et al. Descriptive epidemiological features of bronchiolitis in a population-based cohort. *Pediatrics.* 2008;122(6):1196–1203.
8. Miller EK et al. Viral etiologies of infant bronchiolitis, croup, and upper respiratory illness during four consecutive years. *Pediatr Infect Dis J.* 2014;32(9):950–955.
9. Martinez FD et al. Asthma and wheezing in the first six years of life. *N Engl J Med.* 1995;332:133–138.
10. Morgan WJ et al. Outcome of asthma and wheezing in the first 6 years of life: follow-up through adolescence. *Am J Resp Crit Care Med.* 2005;172(10):1253–1258.

32

Preventing Early-Onset Neonatal Group B Streptococcal Disease

MICHAEL LEVY

The results of this study demonstrate the efficacy of selective intrapartum chemoprophylaxis against early-onset neonatal group B streptococcal disease.

—BOYER AND GOTOFF[1]

Research Question: Does intrapartum antibiotic prophylaxis prevent early-onset neonatal Group B streptococcal disease?[1]

Funding: National Institutes of Health.

Year Study Began: 1979

Year Published: 1986

Study Location: The obstetric clinics of the Michael Reese Hospital and Medical Center in Chicago, an HMO, and private obstetricians' offices.

Who Was Studied: Pregnant women, and the infants of those women, with positive Group B streptococcus (GBS) cultures from vaginal or rectal specimens. Subjects had either premature labor prior to 37 weeks gestation, or prolonged rupture of membranes >12 hours, since those are sepsis risk factors.

Who Was Excluded: Women with penicillin allergy, those receiving other antibiotics, and those with intrapartum temperature greater than 37.5°C.

How Many Patients: 180 women and their 185 newborn infants were randomized. A total of 20 women and their 21 infants were later excluded due to intrapartum fever, randomization errors, or incomplete data. There was also a nonrandomized group of 1,648 women and their 1,658 infants.

Study Overview: See Figure 32.1 for a summary of the study design.

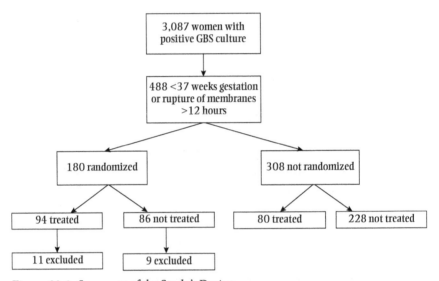

Figure 32.1 Summary of the Study's Design.

Study Intervention: Intrapartum IV ampicillin, 2 grams for the first dose, and then 1 gram every four hours until delivery.

Follow Up: Patients were followed until the results of postpartum cultures were known, and the women's postpartum clinical courses were followed.

Endpoints: Infants were tested for colonization of "surface" sites (external auditory canal, throat, gastric contents, umbilicus, and rectum), and bacteremia. The women were tested for postpartum vaginal group B streptococcal colonization and postpartum illness (temperature > 37.5°C). A primary outcome was not specified.

RESULTS

- Early-onset GBS disease was seen in 5 babies (6.3%) in the randomized control group and in 7 babies (3.1%) in the nonrandomized control group.
- One of the infected infants from the randomized control group died (1.3%).
- In both the randomized and nonrandomized patients, there were no cases of neonatal early-onset GBS disease ($P < 0.001$) or obstetrical infections in the treatment groups.
- 40 of 79 infants (50.6%) in the randomized control group had at least one positive surface culture, compared to 8 of 85 infants (9.4%) in the randomized treatment group ($P < 0.001$).
- Adverse effects were seen in one mother in the treatment group who developed urticaria.

Criticisms and Limitations: The exclusion of 20 women, including 13 with intrapartum fever, may have introduced attrition bias. These women and their babies may have been most likely to be infected, and they were not included in the analysis. No participants in the study, including outcome assessors, were blinded, which may have introduced detection bias. The study excluded women with full-term babies whose membranes were ruptured fewer than 12 hours, so the results might not be generalizable to those patients.

Other Relevant Studies and Information:

- This was the first study to demonstrate a decrease in early-onset neonatal GBS disease with intrapartum antibiotic prophylaxis. Since this study there have been few subsequent randomized-controlled trials examining the efficacy of intrapartum antibiotics for prevention of neonatal GBS disease.[2]
- The incidence of early-onset GBS disease decreased from 1.7 per 1,000 live births in 1993 to 0.6 per 1,000 live births in 1998.[3] While not necessarily causal, this trend was associated with the publishing of guidelines recommending intrapartum antibiotics.
- Antibiotic prophylaxis for laboring women who have had a positive GBS culture during pregnancy is now the standard of care in the United States[4] and many other countries.
- To date, there has not been an observed increase in resistant strains of GBS or other organisms that cause early-onset neonatal sepsis, and the incidence of sepsis due to non-GBS pathogens remains stable.[4]

Summary and Implications: This was the first major study to demonstrate that intrapartum antibiotic prophylaxis decreases early-onset neonatal GBS disease. Current guidelines recommend antibiotic prophylaxis for all women in labor who have had a positive GBS culture during pregnancy. After implementation of treatment guidelines, the incidence of GBS disease decreased by 65% over a 5-year period, and there has not been a concurrent increase in early-onset sepsis due to other pathogens, nor a substantial rise in antibiotic resistance.

CLINICAL CASE: PREVENTING EARLY-ONSET GBS DISEASE

Case History:
You are asked by the obstetrical team to meet a woman who is in labor and soon to deliver her first child. Her doctor has recommended intrapartum ampicillin due to a positive GBS culture late in this pregnancy. She wonders if the benefits outweigh the risks, noting a friend who has a penicillin allergy. She also asks, "Why do I need antibiotics if I don't feel sick?"

Suggested Answer:
This patient has raised some significant and common concerns. You may explain to her that GBS, like many other bacteria, can live on our bodies without causing any illness. GBS is unique in that it sometimes causes serious illnesses in newborns. Infection in babies is much less likely when mothers receive antibiotics in labor. This benefit appears to come without the risk of antibiotic resistance or more infections with other bacteria. With regard to her question about allergic reactions, you might tell her that anaphylaxis with intrapartum antibiotics is extremely rare, especially in a person without previous penicillin allergy, and her doctors will be closely monitoring her for any reaction.

References

1. Boyer KM, Gotoff SP. Prevention of early-onset neonatal group B streptococcal disease with selective intrapartum chemoprophylaxis. *N Engl J Med.* 1986;314(26):1665–1669.
2. Ohlsson A, Shah VS. Intrapartum antibiotics for known maternal Group B streptococcal colonization. *Cochrane Database Syst Rev.* 2014;6:CD007467.

3. Schrag SJ, Zywicki S, Farley MM, et al. Group B streptococcal disease in the era of intrapartum antibiotic prophylaxis. *N Engl J Med.* 2000;342(1):15–20.

4. Verani JR, Mcgee L, Schrag SJ. Prevention of perinatal group B streptococcal disease—revised guidelines from CDC, 2010. *MMWR Recomm Rep.* 2010;59(RR-10):1–36.

SECTION 10

Neonatology

33

Apgar Scoring of Infants at Delivery

MICHAEL LEVY

The purpose of this paper is the reestablishment of simple, clear classification of "grading" of newborn infants which can be used as a basis for discussion and comparison of the results of obstetric practices, types of maternal pain relief and the effects of resuscitation.

—Apgar[1]

Research Question: Can the status of a newborn be described quickly and objectively, and can that description be used to predict outcomes?[1]

Year Published: 1953

Study Location: The Presbyterian Hospital in New York.

Who Was Studied: Liveborn babies during a 7½-month period.

Who Was Excluded: Infants who did not have scoring performed, or for whom the charts were unavailable.

How Many Patients: 1,021

Study Overview: Virginia Apgar was an obstetrical anesthesiologist who sought to describe objectively the status of infants at birth as a way to examine obstetric and anesthetic practices and effects of resuscitation. She began by listing objective signs she felt described a newborn at delivery. She chose five that she felt to be useful and easy to determine. These became the components of the Apgar score (see Table 33.1).

Table 33.1. COMPONENTS OF THE APGAR SCORE

	Apgar score		
	0	1	2
Heart rate	None	<100	100–140
Respiratory effort	Apneic	Irregular or shallow	Breathing or crying
Reflex irritability	None	Reduced	Grimace, sneeze, or cough
Muscle tone	Flaccid	Decreased	Good tone, spontaneously flexed arms and legs
Color	Cyanosis	Acrocyanosis	Entirely pink

Dr. Apgar then looked for factors such as mode of delivery and type of anesthesia that might be associated with lower scores.

RESULTS

- Babies born by spontaneous vaginal or low forceps delivery had higher average scores, 8.4, than babies born by all other methods, which averaged less than 7.0 each.
- Among babies born by cesarean section, those for whom spinal anesthesia was used had an average score of 8.0 (N = 83) while those exposed to general anesthesia averaged 5.0 (N = 54). The study did not account for confounding factors.
- A low 1-minute Apgar score was a predictor of neonatal mortality (Table 33.2).:

Table 33.2. MORTALITY RATE BY APGAR SCORE

Apgar Score	Number	% Mortality
8–10	774	0.1
3–7	182	1.1
0–2	65	13.8

Criticisms and Limitations:

- Fewer than half of babies born during the study period were scored. The author states that most of the deliveries for which the chart was missing were low-risk deliveries. We also know nothing about the 712 live births that were not scored.
- The data were not analyzed statistically and we are left to our intuition to judge the significance of the effect sizes seen.

Additional Information:

- Most institutions added 5-minute scores after they were shown to correlate more closely with mortality.[2]
- A retrospective cohort study that included 132,228 term infants showed increased neonatal death when the 5-minute Apgar score was 0–3 (relative risk = 1460) or 4–6 (relative risk = 53) compared to infants with scores of 7–10.[3]
- Low 5-minute Apgar scores do not correlate closely with neurologic outcomes. In one cohort of 49,000 infants followed for 7 years, 73% of those who developed cerebral palsy had 5-minute Apgar scores ≥7. Eighty-eight percent of children with Apgar scores of 0–3 at 10 minutes who survived did not have cerebral palsy.[4]
- Shortly after the instrument's development, two pediatricians developed a mnemonic to remember the components of the score using the letters of Dr. Apgar's name[5]:
  - **A**ppearance (color)
  - **P**ulse (heart rate)
  - **G**rimace (reflex irritability)
  - **A**ctivity (muscle tone)
  - **R**espiratory effort
- Apgar scores are not used to dictate resuscitation since resuscitative efforts must be initiated before 1 minute of life.

Summary and Implications: The status of a newborn infant can be described quickly and objectively in the delivery room. Some factors such as mode of delivery and type of anesthesia may help predict which babies will have lower scores. Very low scores are predictive of neonatal mortality.

CLINICAL CASE: APGAR SCORING
OF INFANTS AT DELIVERY

Case History:
You are called in the middle of the night to attend the unplanned cesarean section delivery of a full-term infant under general anesthesia. What is the significance of these historical risk factors, and how would you prepare for the resuscitation?

Suggested Answer:
Babies born by cesarean section under general anesthesia have, on average, lower Apgar scores than babies born by other modes or by cesarean section using regional anesthesia. Apgar scores do not dictate resuscitation, but low scores do describe infants who may need intervention, and are associated with risk of neonatal mortality. In this case it would be prudent to ensure backup is available in case the infant requires significant resuscitation. This would include having a sufficient number of providers available dedicated to the baby, and having neonatology ready if possible.

References

1. Apgar V. A proposal for a new method of evaluation of the newborn infant. *Curr Res Anesth Analg.* 1953;32(4):260–267.
2. Finster M, Wood M. The Apgar score has survived the test of time. *Anesthesiology.* 2005;102(4):855–857.
3. Casey BM, Mcintire DD, Leveno KJ. The continuing value of the Apgar score for the assessment of newborn infants. *N Engl J Med.* 2001;344(7):467–471.
4. Nelson KB, Ellenberg JH. Apgar scores as predictors of chronic neurologic disability. *Pediatrics.* 1981;68(1):36–44.
5. Butterfield J, Covey MJ. Practical epigram of the Apgar score. *JAMA.* 1962;181:143.

34

Prophylactic Treatment with Human Surfactant in Extremely Preterm Infants

MICHAEL LEVY

> *The incidence of neonatal death due to the respiratory distress syndrome was much lower, and bronchopulmonary dysplasia ... was decreased among surfactant-treated infants.*
>
> —MERRITT ET AL.[1]

Research Question: Does prophylactic administration of human surfactant to premature infants (24–29 weeks gestation with an immature phospholipid profile) at birth prevent respiratory distress syndrome (RDS), bronchopulmonary dysplasia (BPD), and neonatal death?[1]

Funding: National Institutes of Health, General Clinical Research Center, March of Dimes, Food and Drug Administration, Joan B. Kroc Foundation, Finnish Academy, and the Sigrid Juselius Foundation.

Year Published: 1986

Study Location: University of California–San Diego Medical Center and Children's Hospital, University of Helsinki, Finland.

Who Was Studied: Infants born at 24–29 weeks gestation with an immature phospholipid profile (lecithin/sphingomyelin ratio < 2.0 and absence of phosphatidylglycerol) measured in amniotic fluid before delivery or in pharyngeal or tracheal aspirate after delivery.

Who Was Excluded: Neonates with a mature phospholipid profile, evidence of malformation or diseases that affect lung development, sepsis in the mother, oligohydramnios with rupture of membranes beyond 3 weeks, or >48 hours of betamethasone treatment.

How Many Patients: 60

Study Overview: See Figure 34.1 for a summary of the study design.

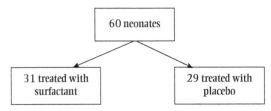

Figure 34.1. Summary of the Study's Design.

Study Intervention: A single dose of human surfactant, injected into the trachea via endotracheal tube immediately after birth.

Follow-Up: Neonates were followed until death or NICU discharge.

Endpoints: The primary outcomes were survival at 28 days with or without bronchopulmonary dysplasia, and death before 28 days. Additional outcomes were ventilator requirements and complications, and duration of NICU admission.

RESULTS

- The surfactant-treated group had significantly lower mortality, BPD, ventilator-associated complications, and duration of NICU stay (see Table 34.1).
- Surfactant-treated infants had significantly lower ventilator requirements including positive end-expiratory pressure, respiratory rate, FiO_2, and mean airway pressure.
- There were no differences between the two groups in the incidence of patent ductus arteriosus, infection, necrotizing enterocolitis, and intraventricular hemorrhage.

- The study was stopped early because of the decreased mortality and morbidity.

Table 34.1. SUMMARY OF THE STUDY'S KEY FINDINGS

	NUMBER OF NEONATES		
	Surfactant Group (n = 31)	Control Group (n = 29)	P value
Death ≤28 days	5 (16%)	15 (52%)	<0.001
Survival with BPD	5 (19%)	9 (62%)	<0.001
Pneumothorax	2 (6%)	7 (24%)	<0.02
Pulmonary interstitial emphysema	1 (3%)	14 (48%)	<0.001
Mean NICU days among survivors	70	122	<0.015

Criticisms and Limitations:

- All infants were immediately intubated and conventionally ventilated. Since that approach is no longer the standard of care, it raises the question of whether surfactant would still be beneficial in the setting of current treatment practices.
- Lecithin/sphingomyelin ratios are no longer assayed routinely, reducing the ability of clinicians to identify individuals most likely to benefit from surfactant therapy.
- The authors do not define BPD, and the definition has evolved since this study was published.

Other Relevant Studies and Information:

- Prophylactic surfactant has been shown to reduce mortality when compared to rescue surfactant, or surfactant administration after RDS is diagnosed.[2]
- A less invasive approach, the technique of intubation, surfactant, and extubation (INSURE), results in reduced ventilator and oxygen requirements compared with rescue surfactant.[2]
- Another less invasive strategy, early use of continuous positive airway pressure (CPAP) with selective surfactant, results in lower rates of mortality and BPD.[3,4]
- The AAP recommends considering using CPAP immediately after birth with selective surfactant administration as an alternative to routine prophylactic surfactant.[2,3]

Summary and Implications: This study was pivotal in establishing the utility of early surfactant administration to appropriately selected extremely preterm infants. When using conventional ventilation techniques, prophylactic surfactant reduces morbidity and mortality compared to placebo. Newer strategies, such as prophylactic surfactant with early extubation or noninvasive ventilation with selective surfactant, may provide even more benefit.

CLINICAL CASE: PROPHYLACTIC SURFACTANT FOR A PRETERM INFANT

Case History:
As the hospital pediatrician on call you are asked to consult on a woman who is about to deliver prematurely at 28 weeks gestation. She is upset and anxious, and concerned specifically about breathing problems that her newborn might have. She tells you of a family member who was born prematurely in the 1980s and died because of "immature lungs."

Suggested Answer:
Compared to 30 years ago, neonatologists have much greater knowledge of the causes of and treatments for respiratory distress syndrome, which was the likely diagnosis in her family member. Surfactant replacement with less invasive ventilation will considerably reduce her infant's chances of death and respiratory complications.

References

1. Merritt TA, Hallman M, Bloom BT, et al. Prophylactic treatment of very premature infants with human surfactant. *N Engl J Med.* 1986;315(13):785–790.
2. Polin RA, Carlo WA. Surfactant replacement therapy for preterm and term neonates with respiratory distress. *Pediatrics.* 2014;133(1):156–163.
3. Respiratory support in preterm infants at birth. *Pediatrics.* 2014;133(1):171–174.
4. Rojas-Reyes MX, Morley CJ, Soll R. Prophylactic versus selective use of surfactant in preventing morbidity and mortality in preterm infants. *Cochrane Database Syst Rev.* 2012;3:CD000510.

Nephrology

35

Oral versus Initial Intravenous Antibiotics for Urinary Tract Infection in Young Febrile Children

MICHAEL LEVY

Our study showed equivalent efficacy of oral cefixime and IV cefotaxime for treatment of young children with fever and [urinary tract infection].
—Hoberman et al.[1]

Research Question: Is oral antibiotic therapy alone as safe and effective as initial treatment with IV followed by oral antibiotics in young children with fever and urinary tract infection (UTI)?[1]

Funding: The Biomedical Research Support Grant Program, Division of Research Resources, the General Clinical Research Center Grants at Children's Hospital of Pittsburgh, and Children's Hospital, Boston, both from the National Institutes of Health, Bethesda, MD, and by Lederle/Wyeth-Ayerst Laboratories.

Year Study Began: 1992

Year Published: 1999

Study Location: Children's Hospital of Pittsburgh, Columbus Children's Hospital, Fairfax Hospital for Children, and Children's Hospital Boston.

Who Was Studied: Children aged 1–24 months with fever (temperature ≥38.3°C) and UTI. UTI was suspected if there was pyuria (≥10 white blood cells/cubic millimeter in uncentrifuged urine) and bacteriuria (≥1 Gram-negative rod/10 oil immersion fields in a Gram-stained smear of uncentrifuged urine). A UTI was defined as ≥50,000 colony-forming units per mL of a single pathogen in a catheterized specimen.

Who Was Excluded: Children with a negative urine culture, cephalosporin allergy, Gram-positive cocci on urine microscopy, unequivocal alternative source for fever, a history of UTI or urinary tract abnormalities, an underlying chronic disease, and those who had received systemic antibiotics within 48 hours of presentation. Three children were deemed too ill and not randomized.

How Many Subjects: 421 children were eligible; 309 were enrolled and had a positive urine culture.

Study Overview: See Figure 35.1 for a summary of the study's design.

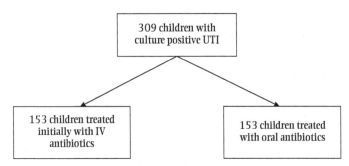

Figure 35.1 Summary of the Study's Design.

Study Intervention: Children were randomized to receive either 14 days of oral cefixime, or IV cefotaxime for 3 days or until afebrile for 24 hours (whichever was longer), followed by completion of a 14-day course with oral cefixime. All children had a ^{99m}Tc-dimercaptosuccinic acid (DMSA) renal scan within 48 hours of study entry.

Follow-Up: 6 months.

Endpoints: Short-term outcomes included sterilization of the urine and defervescence. Long-term outcomes included incidence of reinfection and incidence and extent of renal scarring on DMSA scan at 6 months.

RESULTS

- Repeat urine culture was sterile in all children (291) for whom a repeat culture was available within 24 hours of starting antibiotics.
- Defervescence occurred at 24.7 hours in the oral group, and 23.9 hours in the IV group ($P = 0.76$).
- Symptomatic reinfection occurred at a similar rate in each group (4.6% in the oral antibiotic group, 7.2% in the IV antibiotic group; $P = 0.28$).
- No statistically significant difference was noted in the incidence and extent of renal scarring between the two treatment groups (9.8% in the oral antibiotic group, 7.2% in the IV antibiotic group; $P = 0.21$). This association held true when analyzing only children who had acute pyelonephritis, defined as areas of decreased uptake on DMSA scan without loss of renal contours at presentation.
- Compliance, defined as detectable cefixime in the urine at follow-up, was similar for both treatment groups, though the numbers are not given.

Criticisms and Limitations:

- All but one of the isolated pathogens were sensitive to third-generation cephalosporins. Results may not be generalizable to other antibiotics, or other regions with different resistance patterns of urinary pathogens.
- Most children found to have vesicoureteral reflux when the voiding cystourethrogram was obtained at 4–6 weeks were started on antimicrobial prophylaxis. This may have had an impact on long-term outcomes independent of the initial treatment.

Other Relevant Studies and Information:

- Two similar studies have since shown no difference in incidence of renal scarring at 6–8 months[2] and at 12 months[3] in children as young as 1 month treated initially with IV antibiotics compared to those treated with only oral antibiotics. These studies also showed no difference in time to defervescence.

- The clinical practice guideline from the AAP[4] states that initial treatment with oral or IV antibiotics are equally efficacious and recommends oral antibiotics for nontoxic children who are able to tolerate oral intake. This guideline does not apply to children younger than 2 months. A subsequent Cochrane Review[5] also supported this recommendation.
- A retrospective review of neonates 1–31 days old admitted to the hospital for UTI showed no treatment failures or recurrences.[6] These neonates were treated with IV antibiotics for a median duration of 4 days.
- A retrospective cohort study of infants less than 6 months old with UTI found no difference in treatment failure at 30 days when given an initial short course (≤3 days) of IV antibiotics versus a longer course.[7] Of these infants, 3,383 were <1 month old.[8]

Summary and Implications: Children and infants older than 2 months with fever and UTI may be treated with oral antibiotics alone. When compared to children who initially received IV antibiotics, there is no difference in recurrence or subsequent renal scarring. This means that many children who previously would have been admitted to the hospital are now treated as outpatients. While not included in most studies or the clinical practice guidelines, there is evidence to suggest that a short duration of IV antibiotics followed by oral therapy to complete the course may be safe for infants <2 months old.

CLINICAL CASE: ORAL VERSUS INITIAL INTRAVENOUS ANTIBIOTICS FOR URINARY TRACT INFECTION

Case History:
You are seeing a 6-month-old uncircumcised boy in an urgent care clinic. He presents with a fever of 38.5°C and vomiting. A urinalysis is suspicious for UTI, and a urine culture is sent. How will you deliver the initial dose of antibiotics? Does this child require hospital admission?

Suggested Answer:
Multiple studies in children as young as 1 month have shown that a course of antibiotics using only oral agents is as effective as a course using initial IV antibiotics with regards to multiple outcomes. An outpatient course of oral therapy may be considered. However, this child is vomiting, so you must also consider if he will tolerate the oral medication. In this case, a starting dose of an oral cephalosporin may be appropriate while watching the child also tolerate oral fluids. If unable to do so, a hospital admission may be warranted until he is able to tolerate oral antibiotics.

References

1. Hoberman A, Wald ER, Hickey RW, et al. Oral versus initial intravenous therapy for urinary tract infections in young febrile children. *Pediatrics.* 1999;104(1 Pt 1):79–86.
2. Bocquet N, Sergent Alaoui A, Jais JP, et al. Randomized trial of oral versus sequential IV/oral antibiotic for acute pyelonephritis in children. *Pediatrics.* 2012;129(2):e269–275.
3. Montini G, Toffolo A, Zucchetta P, et al. Antibiotic treatment for pyelonephritis in children: multicentre randomised controlled non-inferiority trial. *BMJ.* 2007;335(7616):386.
4. Roberts KB. Urinary tract infection: clinical practice guideline for the diagnosis and management of the initial UTI in febrile infants and children 2 to 24 months. *Pediatrics.* 2011;128(3):595–610.
5. Strohmeier Y, Hodson EM, Willis NS, Webster AC, Craig JC. Antibiotics for acute pyelonephritis in children. *Cochrane Database Syst Rev.* 2014;7:CD003772.
6. Magín EC, García-García JJ, Sert SZ, Giralt AG, Cubells CL. Efficacy of short-term intravenous antibiotic in neonates with urinary tract infection. *Pediatr Emerg Care.* 2007;23(2):83–86.
7. Brady PW, Conway PH, Goudie A. Length of intravenous antibiotic therapy and treatment failure in infants with urinary tract infections. *Pediatrics.* 2010; 126(2):196–203.
8. Schroeder AR, Ralston SL. Intravenous antibiotic durations for common bacterial infections in children: when is enough enough? *J Hosp Med.* 2014;9(9):604–609.

Identifying Children with Minimal Change Disease

JEREMIAH DAVIS

... the prediction that a child with the primary nephrotic syndrome who responds to intensive steroid treatment has [MCD] is quite accurate....
—INTERNATIONAL STUDY OF KIDNEY DISEASE
IN CHILDREN (ISKDC)

Research Question: For children with nephrotic syndrome, does a favorable response to prednisone help to confirm a diagnosis of minimal change disease (MCD)?[1]

Funding: National Institutes of Health Research Grant 1 RO1 AM18234, Kidney Foundation of New York, Kidney Disease Institute of the State of New York, Kidney Foundation of the Netherlands, National Kidney Research Foundation (United Kingdom), and the John Rath Foundation.

Year Study Began: 1967

Year Study Published: 1981

Study Location: 24 international sites including North and Central America, Europe, Asia, and Israel.

Who Was Studied: Children between 16 weeks and 15 years of age presenting with nephrotic syndrome between January 1967 and April 1976. Participants had hypoalbuminemia (≤2.5 g/dL), overnight urine protein excretion ≥40 mg/hour/m², and a renal biopsy.

Who Was Excluded: Patients formerly treated with immunosuppressive medications (steroid or cytotoxic), or who were diagnosed with any other systemic disease linked to nephrotic syndrome, were excluded. Fifty of the original participants were excluded due to incomplete data collection, and 10 of these were directed to a therapeutic trial after diagnosis with membranoproliferative glomerulonephritis.

How Many Patients: 521

Study Overview: See Figure 36.1 for a summary of the study's design.

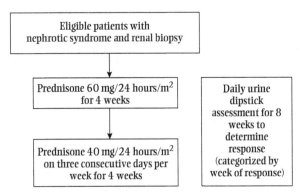

Figure 36.1 Summary of the Study's Design.

Determination of Patient Outcome: Patients were followed with daily urine dipstick assessments. A reduction in proteinuria from baseline to "0 to trace" (4 mg/hour/m²) for 3 days in a row was considered a response to treatment. Participants were followed for a total of 8 weeks.

RESULTS

- 93.1% of those patients with biopsy-proven MCD responded to steroid treatment; however, among all patients who failed to respond to steroid treatment, approximately one-quarter (24.3%) had MCD by biopsy.

- For all nephrotic syndrome causes, 78.1% of patients responded to steroid therapy. Individuals with a biopsy diagnosis of MCD, focal global glomerular obsolescence with tubular atrophy, diffuse mesangial hypercellularity, or unclassified disease had a >50% response rate.
- Overall 93.8% of all steroid responders met outcome criteria by the fourth week of study (reduction in proteinuria to "0 to trace" for 3 days in a row; Figure 36.2).
- Among children ≤6 years of age, 87% of those with nephrotic syndrome had a biopsy diagnosis of MCD ($P < 0.05$ vs. older children) while only 53.2% of children >6 years of age had a biopsy diagnosis of MCD. When divided by response and age (Table 36.1), 23/363 (6.3%) with MCD ≤6 years of age and 2/363 (0.6%) with MCD >6 years of age failed to respond to empiric steroid therapy. Among nonresponders >6 years of age, only 2/55 (3.6%) had biopsy-proven MCD.

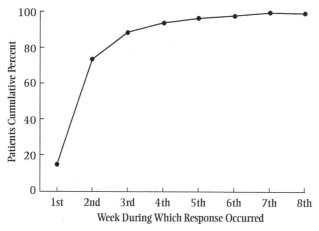

Figure 36.2. Cumulative Distribution of Time to Response for Initial Responders.

Table 36.1 RESPONSE TO STEROID BY AGE AND UNDERLYING NEPHROTIC SYNDROME CAUSE

Group	Patients with MCD (%)	Patients with Other Cause (%)
Responders ≤6 years (n = 284)	266 (93.7)	18 (6.3)
Responders >6 years (n = 84)	72 (85.7)	12 (14.3)
Nonresponders ≤6 years (n = 48)	23 (47.9)	25 (52.1)
Nonresponders >6 years (n = 55)	2 (3.6)	53 (96.4)

Criticisms and Limitations: While this study provides insightful information, it does not directly compare outcomes between children who received a renal biopsy versus those who didn't; thus it remains unclear whether confirmation of patient's diagnosis with renal biopsy will improve outcomes. Given the different rates of renal disease in various ethnic populations, a description of the background patient gender, race, and geographic locations would be insightful.

Other Relevant Studies and Information:

- Much of the methodology governing this study is described in additional publications from the ISKDC.[2-4] In particular, a study looking at clinical and laboratory correlates for predicting underlying nephrotic syndrome etiology showed much confounding in clinical decision making, thus raising the importance of using response to treatment as a helpful diagnostic correlate.[5]
- The ISKDC's findings in this article were corroborated by a smaller cohort (145 children) studied in the United Kingdom that demonstrated a similar overall rate of MCD (76.5%).[6]
- Due to concerns in adult patients about a rising incidence of focal segmental glomerulosclerosis (FSGS), investigators in Kansas City retrospectively looked at MCD and FSGS incidence in their local population (148 patients); they found a substantially smaller percentage of children (52.7%) with MCD and a much higher fraction with FSGS (23%), compared to the ISKDC article.[7] The authors point out differing background rates of renal disease in their geographic and ethnic population and reinforce the limitations of the ISKDC study group when extrapolating findings to other populations.
- The US Children's Nephrotic Syndrome Consensus Conference published guidelines in 2009 recommending that children <12 years of age with nephrotic syndrome be treated initially with steroids, rather than routinely undergoing kidney biopsy. For those ≥12 years, or with steroid-resistant nephrotic syndrome, biopsy should be performed.[8]

Summary and Implications: The ISKDC found that among children with nephrotic syndrome, a response to steroids is highly predictive of biopsy-confirmed MCD. Still, response to steroids is neither completely sensitive nor specific. Based on the results of this and related studies, many nephrologists defer renal biopsy in children with nephrotic syndrome until children have first received a trial of steroids.

CLINICAL CASE: NEPHROTIC SYNDROME IN CHILDHOOD

Case History:

A 4-year-old male presents to your clinic due to parental concern for swelling; his mother relates that over the past week she's noticed his eyelids looking "puffy" bilaterally, but denies any redness, discharge, sneezing, or congestion. She also notes that his legs look chubbier to her and she reports that his urine has a frothy appearance. On office laboratory testing you find that his albumin is low at 1.8 mg/dL and his urine dipstick has 4+ protein notable; his blood pressure is mildly elevated for age but does not meet hypertensive urgency status.

Based on the results of this study, what would be your next step?

Suggested Answer:

Based on the ISKDC's cohort, this patient with nephrotic syndrome who is <6 years old has about a 77% chance that MCD is the underlying etiology; since laboratory and clinical features are not reliable in confirming this, a trial of prednisone for both therapeutic and diagnostic purposes is reasonable. Close follow-up with repeated urinalysis can help confirm response. If he responds, he is 93.7% likely to have MCD, given that only 6.3% of responders in his age group had an alternate etiology. If he does not respond, there is still a nearly 1 out of 2 chance he has MCD, although alternate diagnoses become increasingly likely as well. For his age, the parents can be reassured that most likely he has MCD, and if he responds to steroid treatment he does not warrant additional investigation such as renal biopsy.

References

1. International Study of Kidney Disease in Children. Primary nephrotic syndrome in children. Identification of patients with minimal change nephrotic syndrome from initial response to prednisone. A report of the International Study of Kidney Disease in Children. *J Pediatr.* 1981;98(4):561–564.
2. Abramowitz M et al. Controlled trial of azathioprine in children with nephrotic syndrome: A report of the International Study of Kidney Disease in Children. *Lancet.* 1970;1(7654):959–961.
3. Churg J, Habib R, White RHR. Pathology of the nephrotic syndrome in children: A report for the International Study of Kidney Disease in Children. *Lancet.* 1970;760(1):1299–1301.
4. International Study of Kidney Disease in Children. Prospective controlled trial of cyclophosphamide therapy in children with the nephrotic syndrome. *Lancet.* 1974;2(7878):423–427.

5. International Study of Kidney Disease in Children. Nephrotic syndrome in children: Prediction of histopathology from clinical and laboratory characteristics at time of diagnosis. *Kidney Int.* 1978;13(2):159–165.
6. White RH, Glasgow EF, Mills RJ. Clinicopathological study of nephrotic syndrome in childhood. *Lancet* 1970;1(7661):1353–1359.
7. Srivastava T, Simon SD, Alon US. High incidence of focal segmental glomerulosclerosis in nephrotic syndrome of childhood. *Pediatr Nephrol* 1999;13(1):13–18.
8. Gipson DS et al. Management of childhood onset nephrotic syndrome. *Pediatrics.* 2009;124(2):747–757.

37

Chronic Renal Disease Following Poststreptococcal Glomerulonephritis

JEREMIAH DAVIS

> *These follow-up studies indicate an excellent outcome for patients who recovered clinically from endemic or epidemic [PSGN]....*
>
> —POTTER ET AL.[1]

Research Question: What portion of patients with poststreptococcal glomerulonephritis (PSGN) go on to develop chronic renal abnormalities?[1]

Funding: Ministry of Health of Trinidad and Tobago, the US Public Health Service, Otho S. A. Sprague Memorial Institute.

Year Study Began: 1968

Year Study Published: 1978

Study Location: Trinidad.

Who Was Studied: Randomly selected patients who were affected by epidemic and endemic PSGN in Trinidad between 1965–1969. The diagnosis of PSGN was based on clinical signs of hypertension, hematuria, and edema. Lab abnormalities included azotemia, decreased serum complement concentrations, and positive serology for at least one of the following streptococcal antigens: hyaluronidase, DNAse-B, or streptolysin O.

Who Was Excluded: 15 individuals who were asymptomatic family members of affected patients, but whose routine screening during epidemics revealed laboratory abnormalities.

How Many Patients: 775

Study Overview: See Figure 37.1 for a summary of the study design.

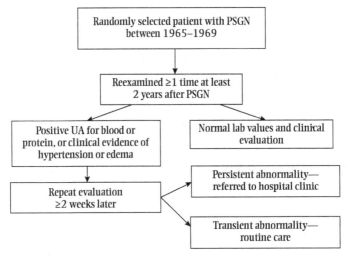

Figure 37.1 Summary of the Study's Design.

Determination of Patient Outcome: At enrollment patients selected for inclusion underwent history and physical examination, including blood pressure measurement, and had a first morning void examined by urinalysis (UA); a second urine sample was collected after 10 minutes in the lordotic position. Any abnormalities led to a referral to the Streptococcal Disease Unit 2 weeks later with an additional first morning specimen and a repeat examination; another lordotic urine sample was obtained. Serum samples were taken for blood urea nitrogen measurement and an assay of $beta_{1c}$ globulin. Abnormalities were considered persistent if both first morning contained protein, or if ≥3 total urine samples contained blood.

Correlation Methods: Chi-square test was used to look for statistical significance in differences between epidemic and endemic patients, age, sex, and race.

RESULTS

- 98.1% of the 775 patients initially randomized to follow-up were successfully examined at least once 2 years after.
- 74% of the included patients had PSGN at ≤10 years of age.
- Excluding lordotic proteinuria, 7.8% of patients had urine abnormalities on at least one examination, whereas only 4.6% had abnormalities on the most recent examination; rates of hematuria, proteinuria, or both are listed in Table 37.1.
- Hypertension was noted in only 11 patients (1.4%) during follow-up.
- Increasing prevalence of hypertension and urine abnormalities was seen with increasing age at PSGN illness; there were no statistically significant differences noted between gender, race, or endemic compared to epidemic patients.
- Of the patients with persistent abnormalities (23 total), 15 were able to be examined at another follow-up, where 12 were found to be abnormal; this cohort was examined two years later where 4 had become normal, 5 were categorized as "transient" abnormalities, and 3 were still persistent; while average follow-up time is not reported, 312 patients were followed up for 5–6 years, and 448 were followed up for 2–4 years.

Table 37.1. Summary of Urine Abnormalities
Noted at Follow-Up Examinations

Abnormality	Any Exam (%)	On Most Recent (%)
Proteinuria alone	22 (2.8%)	11 (1.4%)
Hematuria alone	19 (2.5%)	12 (1.6%)
Proteinuria and hematuria	18 (2.4%)	12 (1.6%)

Criticisms and Limitations: The process of randomization of PSGN patients is not described in any detail; in particular, the "endemic" periods from which certain patients were chosen are not elaborated on in terms of how participants were approached. In addition, patients qualified if they attended at least one follow-up examination; number of assessments for each participant was not equal, and self-selection bias could have resulted since patients choosing to participate in additional follow-up examinations are more likely to perceive themselves as ill. The overall breakdown of streptococcal pharyngitis, skin infections, or other infections is not discussed, limiting the applicability of the study to other populations where streptococcal infection is either endemic or epidemic.

Other Relevant Studies and Information:

- This same cohort was reexamined after 7–12 years of follow-up and again after 12–17 years of follow-up.[2,3] At 7–12 years only 0.8% of the original study group had persistent renal abnormalities (1.1% if 2 additional patients with persistent disease who passed away were included), and 2.3% had hypertension—though this was not significantly higher than baseline rates of hypertension in Trinidad. At 12–17 years 534 of the original patients participated in the study and the incidence of persistent abnormalities rose slightly to 3.5% overall; hypertension was seen in 3.7%, but this was much less than the control group of Trinidadians (11.7%).
- More recently there have been several studies in Venezuela, Australia, and Brazil that have looked at prognosis between 5–18 years after PSGN.[4-6] These studies have supported Potter and colleagues' finding that children were less likely to have severe long-term complications, but also revealed that in certain populations with a background of renal disease, PSGN can lead to more significant sequelae (i.e. Aboriginal populations in Australia).[7]

Summary and Implications: Potter and colleagues found a low incidence of persistent urinary abnormalities or hypertension at least 2 years after PSGN in their population. These data added to a growing body of evidence that better described the clinical course of PSGN, and enabled pediatricians to reserve invasive diagnostic procedures (renal biopsy) and intensive monitoring for those rare children affected by a complicated course of PSGN, or for whom other underlying renal abnormalities were discovered by investigation of PSGN. Based on this improved understanding, most patients now presenting with classic signs and symptoms of PSGN can be monitored as outpatients with simple urine dipstick and blood pressure assessments, and do not undergo renal biopsy.

CLINICAL CASE: URINE ABNORMALITIES FOLLOWING PSGN

Case History:

You are evaluating a 7-year-old female after her discharge from the pediatric hospital for poststreptococcal glomerulonephritis. She was admitted for edema and elevated blood pressures but responded well to diuretics. In your office you obtain a urine dipstick that demonstrates 2+ protein. Her parents are quite concerned and ask if they should return to the hospital. Based on the results of this study, what advice do you give?

Suggested Answer:

Potter et al. provided a large cohort and a relatively long period of follow-up that demonstrated that persistent urinalysis abnormalities can be present in a minority of PSGN patients even years after their initial disease. Other groups have corroborated this. Children are the least likely of all PSGN patients to suffer long-term renal complications, though belonging to a racial or ethnic population with higher rates of renal disease at baseline can make them more susceptible. In addition to reassuring the parents that this finding can be typical of PSGN recovery, you can arrange to continue monitoring this patient's blood pressure and urinalysis findings at routine intervals.

References

1. Potter EV, Abidh S, Sharrett R, et al. Clinical healing two to six years after poststreptococcal glomerulonephritis in Trinidad. *N Engl J Med*. 1978;298(14): 767–772.
2. Nissenson AR, Mayon-White R, Potter EV, et al. Continued absence of clinical renal disease seven to 12 years after poststreptococcal acute glomerulonephritis in Trinidad. *Am J Med*. 1979;67(2):255–262.
3. Potter EV, Lipschultz SA, Abidh S, Poon-King T, Earle DP. Twelve to seventeen-year follow-up of patients with poststreptococcal acute glomerulonephritis in Trinidad. *N Engl J Med*. 1982;307(12):725–729.
4. Rodriguez-Iturbe B. Acute endocapillary glomerulonephritis. In: Davison A et al., ed. *Oxford Textbook of Clinical Nephrology*, 3rd ed. Oxford, England: Oxford University Press; 2005:545–557.
5. Sesso R, Pinto SWL. Five-year follow-up of patients with epidemic glomerulonephritis due to *Streptococcus zooepideicus*. *Nephrol Dial Transplant*. 1005;20(9):1808–1813.
6. White AV, How WE, McCredie DA. Childhood post-streptococcal glomerulonephritis as a risk factor for chronic renal disease in later life. *Med J Aust*. 2001;174(10):492–494.
7. Rodriguez-Iturbe B, Musser JM. The current state of poststreptococcal glomerulonephritis. *J Am Soc Nephrol*. 2008;19(10):1855–1864.

Neurology

38

Antipyretic Agents for Preventing Febrile Seizure Recurrence

NINA SHAPIRO

> *We found that antipyretic agents were ineffective in the prevention of the recurrence of febrile seizures and in the lowering of the fever during an episode that leads to a recurrent seizure.*
>
> —STRENGELL ET AL.[1]

Research Question: Do antipyretic agents reduce the risk of febrile seizure recurrence?

Funding: Special State Grants for Health Research in the Department of Pediatrics and Adolescence at the Oulu University Hospital in Finland.

Year Study Began: 1997

Year Study Published: 2009

Study Location: 5 pediatric hospitals in Finland.

Who Was Studied: Children ages 4 months–4 years who had experienced one prior febrile seizure between January 1, 1997 and December 31, 2003.

Who Was Excluded: Children who had a history of nonfebrile seizures of any type or who had previously used anticonvulsant medication were excluded from the study.

How Many Patients: 231

Study Overview: See Figure 38.1 for a summary of the study's design.

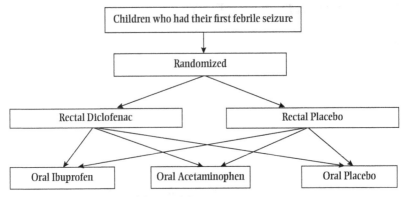

Figure 38.1 Summary of the Study's Design.

Study Intervention: Children who had a previous febrile seizure between January 1, 1997 and December 31, 2003 were randomized to receive a treatment regimen containing a combination of antipyretic agents at their highest recommended doses or placebo every time they had a temperature of 38°C or higher. Patients first received either diclofenac (a prostaglandin inhibitor) (1.5 mg/kg suppository) or placebo rectally for rapid antipyresis followed by oral ibuprofen (10 mg/kg), oral acetaminophen (15 mg/kg), or oral placebo 8 hours later. Oral medication was continued up to 4 times daily for as long as the temperature was greater than 38°C. Patient compliance was maximized by giving families a predesigned sheet to record all febrile episodes, symptoms, and medications given throughout the study period. Study nurses contacted each family at least monthly to ensure appropriate recording of febrile events, and adequate weight-dependent medication dosing. If a child had a nonfebrile seizure, they were discontinued from the study group.

Follow-Up: 2 years.

Endpoints: The primary endpoint was the incidence of febrile seizure recurrence. Secondary endpoints included the effect of the type of first seizure (simple or complex) on the number of recurrences, the maximum temperature of a fever during a febrile episode, the time to first seizure recurrence, the temperature at the time of a febrile seizure, the duration of the febrile seizure, and the administration of extra antipyretic medications.

RESULTS

- All antipyretic agents used in the study were ineffective in the prevention of recurrent febrile seizures and in lowering temperatures during a febrile episode that led to a recurrent febrile seizure. Febrile seizures recurred in 23.5% of patients who received placebo alone and in 23.4% of patients who received any of the antipyretic agents ($P = 0.99$). However, all of the antipyretic agents effectively lowered temperatures in febrile episodes that did not lead to recurrent febrile seizures.
- In all of the treatment groups, the maximum temperature measured during a febrile episode was higher in those febrile episodes that led to a febrile seizure (39.7°C) than in those that did not (38.9°C) ($P < .001$). However, there was no statistical difference between any of the treatment groups in the maximum fever temperature reached during a febrile episode or in the temperature at the time of a seizure.
- Patients receiving rectal diclofenac had a higher fever during the first day of a febrile episode that eventually led to a recurrent febrile seizure and had their seizure recurrences earlier compared to the other treatment groups ($P = 0.01$).
- The majority of febrile seizure recurrences occurred during the first 2 days of a febrile episode and lasted an average of 5.7 minutes.
- There was no statistical difference found in seizure recurrence between children whose initial febrile seizure was simple and those whose initial seizure was complex ($P = 0.38$).

Criticisms and Limitations:

- Caregivers were allowed to administer extra doses of open-label acetaminophen if the temperature of a child rose above 40°C, which might have caused some dilutional bias in the results. Sixty-one percent of study participants received extra antipyretics during the study; however, the distribution of children who received additional antipyretics did not differ among the treatment groups ($P = 0.32$).[1,2]
- The three antipyretic agents used in this trial, diclofenac, ibuprofen, and acetaminophen, have different mechanisms of antipyresis and variable effects on the inhibition of prostaglandin synthesis. In animal studies, it has been observed that some prostaglandins are protective against seizures while some provoke seizures. Should any of these

antipyretic agents provoke seizure, there might again be a dilutional bias when comparing efficacy to placebo alone.[1,2]

Other Relevant Studies and Information:

- The results of this study are supported by the findings in earlier clinical trials that have also concluded that antipyretic agents are ineffective in reducing the risk of febrile seizure recurrence.[2,3]
- There is evidence that antiepileptic medications, either intermittent therapy with diazepam or continuous therapy with phenobarbital, primidone, or valproic acid, reduce the risk of febrile seizure recurrence. However, the Subcommittee on Febrile Seizures of the American Academy of Pediatrics determined that the toxicities of these medications outweigh any potential benefit, and long-term therapy is not recommended. Concordant with this study, the subcommittee also agreed that antipyretics, while improving the comfort of the child, do not reduce fever or prevent febrile-seizure recurrence.[3]

Summary and Implications: Antipyretic agents do not prevent the recurrence of febrile seizures and do not lower temperatures in febrile episodes that lead to a febrile seizure. Antipyretics effectively lower temperatures in febrile episodes that do not produce a febrile seizure, and therefore indications for the use of antipyretic agents should be the same for children with or without a history of febrile seizures.

CLINICAL CASE: RECURRENT FEBRILE SEIZURE

Case History:
The mother of a 3-year-old boy calls you. He has had a recent mild upper respiratory illness, and his temperature rose from 100°F to 104°F in the last hour. She mentioned that 6 months ago, he had a similar illness, and a high fever associated with a seizure. She is anxious, and would like to know how best to minimize the chances of this febrile episode progressing to a febrile seizure.

Suggested Answer:
Based on the article by Strengell et al., use of high-dose, rapid-onset antipyretics have no impact on minimizing the likelihood of a recurrent febrile seizure in a young child with a history of febrile seizures. Despite this, antipyretics (alternating acetaminophen and ibuprofen up to every 3 hours) can still be recommended to help reduce the fever and to make the child more comfortable. Recommending antipyretics is indicated in this situation. However, the patient's mother should be counseled that doing so might have no bearing on her son's fever progressing to a seizure yet again.

References

1. Strengell T, Uhari M, Tarkka R, Uusimaa J, Alen R, Lautala P, Rantala H. Antipyretic agents for preventing recurrences of febrile seizures: randomized controlled trial. *Arch Pediatr Adolesc Med.* 2009;163(9):799–804.
2. Lux AL. Antipyretic drugs do not reduce recurrences of febrile seizures in children with previous febrile seizure. *Evid Based Med.* 2010;15(1):15–6.
3. Steering Committee on Quality Improvement and Management, Subcommittee on Febrile Seizures, American Academy of Pediatrics. Febrile seizures: clinical practice guideline for the long-term management of the child with simple febrile seizures. *Pediatrics.* 2008;121(6):1281–1286.

39

Febrile Seizures and Risk for Epilepsy

ASHAUNTA ANDERSON

In the present study, suspect or abnormal prior [neurological or developmental] status were found to identify a small subgroup of children with febrile seizures who were at high risk for the development of afebrile seizures. In contrast, the majority of children with febrile seizures, those who were normal before any seizure and whose first febrile seizure was not complex, had a rate of subsequent epilepsy that, although higher than for children with no febrile seizures, was still fairly low (11 per 1000, or 1.1 per cent).

—NELSON & ELLENBERG[1]

Research Question: What are the rates and predictors of afebrile seizures in children who have had febrile seizures?[1]

Funding: The National Institute of Neurological and Communicative Disorders and Stroke.

Year Study Began: 1959

Year Study Published: 1976

Study Location: 12 urban teaching hospitals participating in the Collaborative Perinatal Project of the National Institute of Neurological and Communicative Disorders and Stroke.

Who Was Studied: Of the 40,885 children in the Collaborative Perinatal Project with medical records available through 7 years of age, 1,706 experienced a seizure that was:

- The first seizure he or she ever experienced
- Accompanied by fever
- Occurred between 1 month and 7 years of age
- Not symptomatic of recognized acute neurological illness such as meningitis, lead encephalopathy, significant dehydration, and immunization-related seizures

Who Was Excluded: Children with meningitis, lead encephalopathy, significant dehydration, and immunization-related seizures.

How Many Patients: 40,885

Study Overview: See Figure 39.1 for a summary of the study's design.

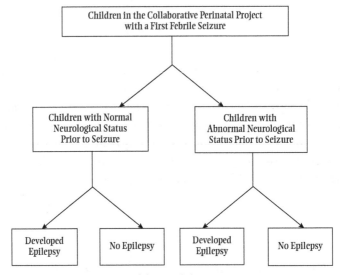

Figure 39.1 Summary of the Study's Design.

Study Intervention: Prior to their first seizure, children's baseline neurological and developmental status was evaluated by standard physical examination at age 4 months, Bayley Scales of Mental and Motor Development at 8 months, and general and neurological examination at 12 months. Medical records were reviewed at ages 4, 8, 12, 18, and 24 months and then annually through age 7 years. Any evidence of epilepsy was noted.

Follow-Up: Children were followed through 7 years of age.

Endpoints: The primary outcome was epilepsy after a first febrile seizure. The study's definition of epilepsy required recurrent afebrile seizures unrelated to an acute neurologic condition. One of the afebrile seizures must have taken place after the age of 48 months.

RESULTS

- Rates of epilepsy were increased when the child's baseline *neurological status was not normal* (12 [normal status] vs. 39 [abnormal status] per 1,000; $P < 0.001$) (see Table 39.1).
- Compared to children with normal baseline neurological status, those with abnormal baseline neurological status had higher rates of epilepsy with each complex feature (i.e., focal features, duration > 15 minutes, or > 1 seizure in 24 hours) of their first febrile seizure.
  - Observed epilepsy rates were low and relatively flat for children with normal baseline neurological status even with a complex first febrile seizure.
  - Among children with normal baseline status, 3 or more seizures indicated higher risk for epilepsy.
- No significant difference in epilepsy rate after a first febrile seizure was found according to:
  - Participating hospital
  - Sex
  - Race (white vs. black)
  - Apgar score
  - Birth weight
- While nearly half of afebrile seizures took place within 1 year of the first febrile seizure, three-quarters occurred within 3 years.

Table 39.1. SUMMARY OF THE STUDY'S KEY FINDINGS

Feature	Number of Children[a]	Epilepsy Rate/ 1,000	Any Afebrile Seizure Rate/1,000
No febrile seizures	39,179	5	9
Febrile seizures			
Prior status normal			
1st febrile seizure simple[b]	1,036	11	17
1st febrile seizure complex	229	20	35
Prior status not normal	290	28	31
1st febrile seizure simple	65	92	123
1st febrile seizure complex			

Adapted from Table 1 of Nelson KB, Ellenberg JH. Predictors of epilepsy in children who have experienced febrile seizures. *N Engl J Med.* 1976;295:1029–1033, which reports the rates of afebrile seizures by the age of 7 years.
[a]Eighty-five children are not included because their prior status was not known, and 1 child is not included because his or her first febrile seizure type was not known.
[b]Simple febrile seizures are those without complex features defined as focal features, duration > 15 minutes, or > 1 seizure in 1 day.

Criticisms and Limitations: Afebrile seizures that occurred after 7 years of age were not captured by the study, so the reported results may be lower than the true rates of epilepsy after febrile seizure. The authors address this limitation by stating the majority of the sample was followed at least 3 years after the first febrile seizure, which is a known peak time interval for seizure recurrence. The authors also state that 13% of the children received antiepileptic medication following their febrile seizures, but distribution across the subgroups and level of seizure control are not specified. Assuming some level of seizure control was achieved for those with the most severe disease, the reported afebrile seizure rates should underreport the true rates for those with greater neurological impairment.

Other Relevant Studies and Information:

- The risk of epilepsy for children with febrile seizures was 6%–7% in studies that followed children into the third decade of life[2-4]; those with shorter follow-up times estimated the risk at 2%–6%.[5,6]
- Risk factors for epilepsy after febrile seizure included complex seizures, prior brain disease, family history of epilepsy, low Apgar scores, number of febrile seizures, and age greater than 3 years at the onset of febrile seizures.[2,3,5,6]
- There is no recommended therapy to prevent the development of epilepsy after simple febrile seizures.
  - The American Academy of Pediatrics does not recommend antiseizure medication for children with 1 or more febrile seizures as the side effects of medication outweigh any benefits.[7]
  - Antipyretic medications are effective to reduce fever, but have not been shown to reduce seizure recurrence.[7]

Summary and Implications: Two percent of children with a first febrile seizure developed epilepsy by 7 years of age. The greatest risk for subsequent afebrile seizures was seen in those with a prior underlying neurological condition or history of a first complex febrile seizure. Most children with a first febrile seizure did not exhibit complex features or baseline neurological problems. Their risk for epilepsy decreased to 1%, but was still higher than that of the general population with no history of febrile seizures (0.5%). Importantly, for this group, repeated febrile seizures were not a risk factor for epilepsy, and antiepileptic drugs may cause more harm in side effects than benefit in seizure reduction.

CLINICAL CASE: FEBRILE SEIZURES AND RISK FOR EPILEPSY

Case History:

A 15-month-old boy presents to the emergency department after losing consciousness and rhythmically twitching his arms and legs for 5 minutes. His mother immediately dialed emergency medical services for transport to the hospital. She reports that he felt warm and was increasingly fussy as the evening progressed. He had a small amount of nasal discharge and a mild cough. He was also less interested in eating, but maintaining normal wet diapers. She denies that the boy has any significant prior medical history, family history, or medication use. On further probing, you learn that the boy does not use words and is not yet walking.

In the emergency department, he is napping in his mother's lap, but begins crying when placed on the examination table. His temperature is elevated to 102°F, but his other vital signs are within expected limits. Aside from a flushed appearance and minimal crust in both nares, his physical examination is unremarkable.

The family is visibly shaken from this experience. What guidance do you offer on the likelihood that this first febrile seizure may be a sign of future epilepsy?

Suggested Answer:

The boy in this scenario has likely experienced a simple febrile seizure, based on the generalized nature of the seizure and duration less than 15 minutes. Twenty-four hours must elapse without a repeat seizure to confirm that he in fact had a simple febrile seizure. These features favor the likelihood that he will not go on to experience 2 or more afebrile seizures (epilepsy). However, it is unusual that he has not produced a word or walked by 15 months of age. This is concerning for developmental delay, which would place him in the category of children without normal neurological status prior to his febrile seizure. According to the study by Nelson and colleagues, 28 out of 1,000 children without normal neurological status who had a first simple febrile seizure went on to develop epilepsy. Therefore, you may counsel the parents that, although his developmental status places him at greater risk for epilepsy, the features of his seizure are favorable. Instead of the baseline half-percent risk in the general population, he still has a low risk of epilepsy after febrile seizure at approximately 3%.

References

1. Nelson KB, Ellenberg JH. Predictors of epilepsy in children who have experienced febrile seizures. *N Engl J Med.* 1976;295:1029–1033.
2. Annegers et al. Factors prognostic of unprovoked seizures after febrile convulsions. *N Engl J Med.* 1987;316(9):493–498.
3. Vestergaard et al. The long-term risk of epilepsy after febrile seizures in susceptible subgroups. *Am J Epidemiol.* 2007;165(8):911–918.
4. Neligan et al. Long-term risk of developing epilepsy after febrile seizures: A prospective cohort study. *Neurology.* 2012;78:1166–1170.
5. Pavlidou et al. Prognostic factors for subsequent epilepsy in children with febrile seizures. *Epilepsia.* 2013;54(12):2101–2107.
6. Verity et al. Risk of epilepsy after febrile convulsions: A national cohort study. *BMJ.* 1991;303:1373–1376.
7. Steering Committee on Quality Improvement and Management, Subcommittee on Febrile Seizures. Febrile seizures: Clinical practice guideline for the long-term management of the child with simple febrile seizures. *Pediatrics.* 2008;121:1281–1286.

40

Seizure Recurrence after First Unprovoked Afebrile Seizure

ASHAUNTA ANDERSON

In this prospective study of children identified at the time of their first unprovoked seizure, the risk of recurrence after 8 years of follow-up is less than 50%.

—SHINNAR ET AL.[1]

Research Question: What is the risk of seizure recurrence after a first unprovoked (no clear proximal insult such as head trauma) afebrile seizure in childhood?[1]

Funding: National Institute of Neurological Disorders and Stroke.

Year Study Began: 1983

Year Study Published: 1996

Study Location: Montefiore Medical Center, Bronx Municipal Hospital Center, North Central Bronx Hospital, or local private practices.

Who Was Studied: Children 1 month to 19 years of age who presented with their first unprovoked afebrile seizure, defined as:

- One or more seizures occurring within 24 hours
- Status epilepticus (seizure lasting longer than 30 minutes or repeated seizures with no return to consciousness for at least 30 minutes)

Who Was Excluded: Children with typical absence seizures, myoclonic seizures, or infantile spasms were excluded. Those with a first generalized tonic-clonic seizure, but a history of absence, myoclonic, or partial seizures were also excluded. Children with a history of provoked seizures such as neonatal, febrile, or posttraumatic seizures were included in the study.

How Many Patients: 407

Study Overview: See Figure 40.1 for a summary of the study's design.

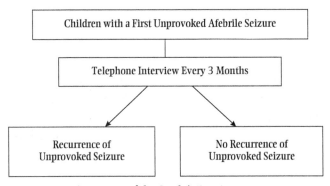

Figure 40.1 Summary of the Study's Design.

Study Intervention: History and physical examination were performed for each enrolled child. If the child had static encephalopathy from birth or a prior neurological insult such as stroke or significant trauma, the presenting seizure was classified as *remote symptomatic*. All other presenting seizures were classified as *cryptogenic*. EEG was performed for most children (94%) and reviewed by study authors who were blinded to outcomes. CT and MR imaging were performed when clinically indicated.

Follow-Up: Seizure recurrence was assessed by telephone interview every 3 months after enrollment for an average of 6.3 years (range = 0.1–10.8 years). Those with repeat unprovoked seizures were evaluated by review of the emergency department record and with an office visit.

Endpoints: The primary outcome was seizure recurrence, which was defined as the occurrence of an unprovoked seizure more than 24 hours after the first seizure.

RESULTS

- Of the 407 children with a first unprovoked afebrile seizure, 171 (42%) had another seizure.
  - The mean time to recurrence was 11.3 months (median 5.7 months).
  - Nearly 90% of seizure recurrences happened within 2 years of the first seizure.
- Children whose initial episode was classified as a remote symptomatic seizure were more likely to have a recurrence than those with a cryptogenic seizure (68% vs. 37% respectively).
- EEG and first unprovoked seizure during sleep versus awake state only predicted seizure recurrence for those with a first cryptogenic seizure (see Table 40.1).
  - Among the 50 children with a first cryptogenic seizure during sleep and an abnormal EEG, seizure recurrence risk was 65% at 5 years.
  - Of the 136 children with a first cryptogenic seizure while awake and a normal EEG, seizure recurrence risk was 21% at 5 years.

Table 40.1. SUMMARY OF THE STUDY'S KEY FINDINGS[a]

Risk Factor	PROPORTIONATE HAZARDS MODEL		
	Rate Ratio	95% CI[b]	*P* Value
Overall Group (N = 407)			
Abnormal EEG	2.1	1.6–3.0	<0.001
Remote symptomatic etiology	1.7	1.2–2.4	0.006
Prior febrile seizures	1.6	1.1–2.3	0.019
Todd's paresis	1.7	1.0–2.9	0.038
Seizure while asleep	1.5	1.1–2.1	0.008
Cryptogenic Cases (N = 342)			
Abnormal EEG	2.5	1.7–3.6	<0.0001
Seizure while asleep	1.7	1.2–2.5	<0.003
Remote Symptomatic Cases (N = 65)			
Prior febrile seizures	2.3	1.2–4.5	<0.02
Age ≤ 3 years	2.4	1.2–4.9	<0.02

[a]Adapted from Table 2 of Shinnar et al. The risk of seizure recurrence after a first unprovoked afebrile seizure in childhood: An extended follow-up. *Pediatrics.* 1996;98:216–225, which reports the risk factors for seizure recurrence using multivariate analysis and a Cox proportional hazards model.
[b]95% confidence interval.

Criticisms and Limitations: These study findings do not apply to children with excluded seizure types. For example, those with absence or myoclonic seizures were excluded because they may have several seizures before they come to medical attention. Therefore, investigators would not be able to comment on recurrence rates after their first seizure. In addition, the children included in this study were followed for an average of 6.3 years, so it is possible that some seizure recurrences beyond the follow-up period may have been missed.

Other Relevant Studies and Information:

- Shinnar and colleagues continued following the group of 407 children and reported a 46% cumulative risk of recurrence 10 years after a first unprovoked seizure.[2]
- The recurrence risk was 54% in 156 children 2 years after a first unprovoked seizure, and:
  - 74% in those with a remote symptomatic etiology
  - 71% with epileptiform patterns on EEG[3]
- In contrast, a study of 119 children with normal neurological exams and a first unprovoked generalized tonic-clonic seizure found an 8-year recurrence risk of 37.7%.[4]
  - Like the study by Shinnar et al, most of the recurrences (87%) took place in the first 2 years.
- Given the low seizure recurrence risk for otherwise healthy children and only short-term seizure reduction with medical therapy, the American Academy of Neurology finds[5,6]:
  - No indication for antiepileptic drugs as a means to prevent the development of epilepsy (2 or more seizures)
  - Antiepileptic drugs should only be used when the benefits of reducing the risk of a second seizure outweigh the side effects of medication
- According to a large retrospective review, emergent neuroimaging is not required in the evaluation of new-onset afebrile seizure unless these high-risk factors are present[7]:
  - Predisposing conditions defined as sickle cell disease, bleeding problems, cerebrovascular disease, cancer, HIV infection, hemihypertrophy, hydrocephaly, closed-head injury, and travel to a cysticercosis-endemic region
  - Focal seizure in a child younger than 33 months old

Summary and Implications: The majority of children who have a first unprovoked seizure will not have a recurrence. If they do have a recurrence, it usually happens within 1–2 years after the first seizure. Cryptogenic etiology, seizure while awake, and normal EEG predict lower recurrence rates.

CLINICAL CASE: FIRST UNPROVOKED AFEBRILE SEIZURE

Case History:
A 5-year-old girl presents to her pediatrician's office to follow up the prior night's emergency department visit for seizure. Her father describes the seizure as a 2-minute period during which his daughter lost consciousness and her limbs stiffened and jerked repeatedly. He states that she did not have a fever, but had experienced several bouts of diarrhea in the preceding days. He denies any preceding trauma, significant past medical history, recent medications, or suspected ingestions.

Upon presentation to the emergency department, she had been sleepy but arousable. Her temperature was normal as were her other vital signs. Her physical exam was unremarkable, including a full neurological exam. She was monitored until she returned to baseline mental status and demonstrated sufficient oral intake. The family was instructed to follow up with neurology and see the pediatrician in the interim.

This morning the girl remains afebrile and alert. She continues to have loose stools, but is drinking lots of fluids and maintaining normal urine output. After a reassuring history and physical exam, what counseling do you offer regarding the likelihood of this girl to experience a repeat seizure?

Suggested Answer:
The girl in this scenario experienced a first unprovoked afebrile seizure. She had no prior history of seizure. She also had none of the insults known to trigger seizure such as fever, head trauma, or toxic ingestion. She was ill with diarrhea, but no electrolyte disturbances were expected given her normal physical examination and sustained oral intake and urine output.

The classification used in the study divides seizures into those that are *remote symptomatic* (due to an earlier neurological insult like static encephalopathy) and all others, called *cryptogenic*. This girl had no significant medical history, so her seizure type is cryptogenic. That means the family may be reassured that she has half the risk of a child who already had some neurological troubles. Only 1 in 3 children like herself go on to have a second seizure. Because she was awake at seizure onset, her risk of a second seizure may even decrease to 1 in 5 if she has a normal EEG. If she did have a second seizure, it would be most likely to happen in the first 2 years after her seizure. Finally, the ultimate management decision rests with the clinician in consultation with the family, but it is unlikely that antiseizure medication will be recommended for this patient.

References

1. Shinnar et al. The risk of seizure recurrence after a first unprovoked afebrile seizure in childhood: An extended follow-up. *Pediatrics*. 1996;98:216–225.

2. Shinnar et al. Predictors of multiple seizures in a cohort of children prospectively followed from the time of their first unprovoked seizure. *Ann Neurol*. 2000;48:140–147.

3. Stroink et al. The first unprovoked, untreated seizure in childhood: A hospital based study of the accuracy of the diagnosis, rate of recurrence, and long-term outcome after recurrence. *J Neurol Neurosurg Psychiatry*. 1998;64:595–600.

4. Bulloche et al. Risk of recurrence after a single, unprovoked, generalized tonic-clonic seizure. *Dev Med Child Neurol*. 1989;31:626–632.

5. Hirtz et al. Practice parameter: Evaluating a first nonfebrile seizure in children. *Neurology*. 2000;55:616–623.

6. Hirtz et al. Practice parameter: Treatment of the child with a first unprovoked seizure. *Neurology*. 2003;60:166–175.

7. Sharma et al. The role of emergent neuroimaging in children with new-onset afebrile seizures. *Pediatrics*. 2003;111(1):1–5.

41

Mortality and Childhood-Onset Epilepsy

ASHAUNTA ANDERSON

Childhood-onset epilepsy was associated with a substantial risk of epilepsy-related death, including sudden, unexplained death. The risk was especially high among children who were not in remission.

—SILLANPÄÄ ET AL.[1]

Research Question: What is the long-term mortality profile associated with childhood-onset epilepsy?[1]

Funding: The Finnish Epilepsy Research Foundation.

Year Study Began: 1964

Year Study Published: 2010

Study Location: The Turku University Hospital, Turku, Finland.

Who Was Studied: Children with epilepsy—defined as two or more unprovoked seizures—who were living in the Turku University Hospital catchment area at the end of 1964 were studied. Included children presented for evaluation from 1961 to 1964 with newly diagnosed epilepsy (61%) or established epilepsy, requiring at least one seizure in the 3 years prior to presentation (39%). Epilepsy was categorized as remote symptomatic when there was preexisting significant neurologic impairment or insult. Otherwise, the epilepsy was considered cryptogenic or idiopathic.

Who Was Excluded: Children with febrile seizures, other acute symptomatic seizures, or a single unprovoked seizure were excluded. Children with an epilepsy diagnosis who were in remission or died prior to 1961 were also excluded.

How Many Patients: 245

Study Overview: See Figure 41.1 for a summary of the study's design.

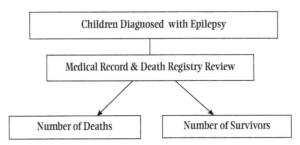

Figure 41.1 Summary of the Study's Design.

Study Intervention: Children received follow-up examinations every 5 years until 2002. Interval review of medical records provided data on the timing of deaths and immediate and underlying causes of death. The Finnish National Death Register was also consulted every 5 years to improve detection of any deaths. Toxicological screening was performed for all who died and autopsy for 70%. All children were followed until death or January 1, 2003 except 5 who migrated out of Finland.

Follow-Up: The median follow-up time was 40 years.

Endpoint: Primary endpoint: Death. Secondary endpoint: Cause of death.

RESULTS

- After a median follow-up time of 40 years, there was a 24% case fatality rate for individuals with childhood-onset epilepsy (see Table 41.1).
- Of the 60 individuals who died, cause of death was attributed to:
  - a neurologic condition or other disease unrelated to epilepsy (43%)
  - an epilepsy-related problem such as sudden, unexplained death in epilepsy (30%), probable or definite seizure (15%), and accidental drowning (10%)
- Higher rates of death occurred in individuals who:
  - were not in 5-year terminal remission (15.9 deaths/1,000 person-years) versus those who were in remission (11.8/1,000 person-years

     for those receiving seizure medication and 1.5/1,000 person-years
     for those not receiving seizure medication); *P* < 0.001
- had remote symptomatic epilepsy (11.1 deaths/1,000 person-
  years) versus those with cryptogenic (2.9/1,000 person-years) or
  idiopathic (3.5/1,000 person-years) epilepsy; *P* <0.001
- When age at onset of epilepsy, prior status epilepticus, type of
  epilepsy, and 5-year terminal remission were included in the
  multivariate model, only 5-year terminal remission significantly
  predicted hazard ratio for death (*P* < 0.007 for all deaths and epilepsy-
  related deaths; *P* < 0.02 for sudden, unexplained deaths).
- Greater detail about the deaths is available in a follow-up article by the
  authors.[2]

Table 41.1. SUMMARY OF THE STUDY'S KEY FINDINGS[a]

Variable	All Children with Epilepsy (N = 245)	Idiopathic or Cryptogenic Epilepsy (N = 122)	Remote Symptomatic Epilepsy[b] (N = 123)
Total Deaths—number	60	15	45
Median Age at Death—years	23	26	21
Number of person-years	8,692	4,638	4,054
Deaths/1,000 person-years[c]			
All	6.9 (5.3–8.9)	3.23 (1.9–5.4)	11.1 (8.3–14.9)
Male	7.33(5.2–10.2)	2.69 (1.2–6)	11.63 (8–16.8)
Female	6.41 (4.4–9.4)	3.74 (1.9–7.2)	10.33 (6.4–16.6)
Remission Status at Time of Death[d]			
Not in remission			
Number/total number of deaths (%)	51/60 (85)	11/15 (73)	40/45 (89)
In remission			
Number/total number of deaths (%)	9/60 (15)	4/15 (27)	5/45 (11)
Receiving medication—number	5	2	3
Not receiving medication—number	4	2	2

[a]Adapted from Table 1 in the study Sillanpää et al. Long-term mortality in childhood-onset epilepsy. *NEJM.* 2010;363:2522–2529.
[b]Remote symptomatic etiology relates epilepsy to a prior significant neurological impairment or insult
[c]Number of deaths per 1,000 person-years, 95% confidence interval.
[d]Remission status at time of death refers to the presence or absence of seizures in the five years prior to death.

Criticisms and Limitations: This study was conducted in a well-characterized Finnish cohort with thorough outcome measures, but the findings may not fully generalize to other countries with different demographics and mortality-related factors. Participants were followed for a median time of forty years, which includes the known peak ages for sudden, unexplained death related to epilepsy. It is likely that the mortality rate would rise with continued follow-up beyond this point, but this may be of diminishing value. The authors note an inherent limitation in the challenge of accurately assessing cause of death after 50 years of age.

Other Relevant Studies and Information:

- A Minnesota-based study of childhood epilepsy with up to 30 years of follow-up found that 16 of 467 children died (3.4%).[3]
  - Fourteen deaths were caused by a disease unrelated to epilepsy and 2 were epilepsy related (1 possible sudden, unexplained death in epilepsy and 1 aspiration event during seizure).
  - Risk factors for death included abnormal cognition, abnormal neurological exam, structural or metabolic etiology for epilepsy, and poorly controlled epilepsy.
- Investigators in Nova Scotia followed 692 children with epilepsy for a median of 14 years and documented 16 deaths (3.8%) using medical and administrative records.[4]
  - The only independent predictor of mortality was functional neurological deficit.
  - Children without a severe neurological deficit had a death rate similar to that of the general population.
- Retrospective review of the death records of 265 children with epilepsy in the United Kingdom revealed cause of death unrelated to epilepsy in about two-thirds of the sample and sudden, unexplained death in less than one-tenth.[5]
  - Sudden, unexplained death was limited to those with documented or presumed symptomatic epilepsy.
  - Unlike the focal study of this chapter, no cases of sudden, unexplained death occurred in children with idiopathic epilepsy.
- A study of over 13,000 children with epilepsy in South Carolina evaluated administrative data from 2000 to 2011 and reported a death rate of 8.8 deaths per 1,000 person-years.[6]
  - While no age, sex, or racial disparities were found for the comparison between children with epilepsy who died and those who survived, non-Hispanic black children, who represented 29% of the state population, accounted for 38% of the children with epilepsy, and 41% of those who died.

Summary and Implications: Childhood-onset epilepsy was associated with a mortality rate that was three times that of the general population after adjustment for age and sex. Absence of five-year terminal remission was the single most important risk factor for both all-cause and epilepsy-related death. However, the study authors do not recommend aggressive treatment based on this finding alone. Further investigation is required to make this determination.

CLINICAL CASE: MORTALITY AND CHILDHOOD-ONSET EPILEPSY

Case History:

An 8-year-old boy with a history of one prior unprovoked seizure was transported to the emergency department actively seizing. He was unconscious, drooling, and rhythmically jerking all four extremities. Repeated doses of antiepileptic medications were administered until the movements ceased. Because he showed signs of increasing respiratory depression, he was intubated for airway protection and admitted to the intensive care unit. He was soon weaned off the ventilator and transferred to the general pediatric ward where you are the receiving physician.

On physical exam, the boy has normal vital signs. He is awake and interactive. The remainder of the exam is also normal, including the neurologic portion. After the exam is complete and the boy is once again settled into bed, the parents ask if they can speak with you privately. They share how their son has been completely healthy with the exception of these two unprovoked seizures. The whole ordeal has been very frightening, and they tearfully admit there were times when they were not sure he would survive. They conclude by asking how likely it is he will die from his seizure disorder. How do you reply to their question?

Suggested Answer:

It is best to sit down with the parents in a quiet place and begin by acknowledging their feelings and concerns. This is not a question that can be answered with 100% accuracy for an individual, but there are some helpful population-based studies. The main study in this chapter does confirm some increased risk of death for children who have epilepsy—up to three times greater than the general population. However, nearly half that risk goes away for children with epilepsy and no other health problems. Other studies have confirmed the finding that otherwise healthy children have little to no increased risk of death attributable to epilepsy. In addition, some epilepsy-related risk factors for death may be mitigated with proper seizure precautions such as taking showers instead of baths. Finally, it is important that the parents are connected to the appropriate clinical and community supports.

References

1. Sillanpää et al. Long-term mortality in childhood-onset epilepsy. *NEJM.* 2010;363:2522–2529.
2. Sillanpää et al. SUDEP and other causes of mortality in childhood-onset epilepsy. *Epilepsy and Behavior.* 2013;28:249–255.
3. Nickels et al. Epilepsy-related mortality is low in children: A 30-year population-based study in Olmstead County, MN. *Epilepsia.* 2012;53(12):2164–2171.
4. Camfield et al. Death in children with epilepsy: A population-based study. *Lancet.* 2002;359:1891–1895.
5. Nesbitt et al. Risk and causes of death in children with a seizure disorder. *Dev Med Child Neurol.* 2012;54:612–617.
6. Selassie et al. Premature deaths among children with epilepsy—South Carolina, 2000–2011. *Morb Mortal Wkly Rep.* 2014;63(44):989–999.

42

Identifying Children with Low-Risk Head Injuries Who Do Not Require Computed Tomography

MICHAEL HOCHMAN, REVISED BY ASHAUNTA ANDERSON

[We] derived and validated highly accurate prediction rules for children at very low risk of [clinically important traumatic brain injuries] for whom CT scans should typically be avoided. Application of these rules could limit CT use, protecting children from unnecessary radiation risks.

—KUPPERMANN ET AL.[1]

Research Question: Is it possible to develop a clinical prediction rule for identifying children at very low risk for clinically important traumatic brain injuries who do not require computed tomography (CT) scans for evaluation?[1]

Funding: The Pediatric Emergency Care Applied Research Network (PECARN), a federally funded organization supported by the United States Health Resources and Services Administration.

Year Study Began: 2004

Year Study Published: 2009

Study Location: 25 emergency departments in the United States.

Who Was Studied: Children younger than 18 presenting to emergency departments within 24 hours of blunt traumatic head injury.

Who Was Excluded: Children with "trivial" injuries such as ground-level falls without signs or symptoms of head injuries aside from scalp lacerations or abrasions, as well as children with penetrating trauma, brain tumors, and "pre-existing neurological disorders." In addition, children with ventricular shunts, bleeding disorders, and Glasgow Coma Scale (GCS) scores under 14 were excluded from this analysis.

How Many Patients: 42,412

Study Overview: See Figure 42.1 for a summary of the study design.

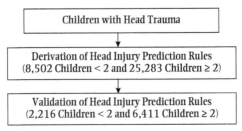

Figure 42.1 Summary of the Study's Design.

Derivation of Prediction Rules: Emergency department physicians interviewed and examined a sample of children with head trauma (the derivation sample) to collect information about each child's history and physical examination findings. This information was collected prior to head imaging (if imaging was performed). The patient information was then correlated with patient outcomes (i.e., whether or not patients were ultimately found to have clinically important traumatic brain injuries [ciTBIs]) to develop prediction rules for assessing brain injury risk.

Validation of Prediction Rules: The prediction rules were then applied to a separate sample of children (the validation sample) presenting with blunt head trauma to assess how well the rules forecasted whether or not these children would ultimately be diagnosed with ciTBI.

Determination of Patient Outcomes: Research coordinators determined which children were ultimately diagnosed with ciTBI by reviewing the medical records of all children admitted to the hospital. In addition, research coordinators conducted telephone interviews with the guardians of all children discharged from the emergency department to identify any children with missed injuries.

ciTBIs were defined as:

- death from traumatic brain injury
- neurosurgery
- intubation for >24 hours
- hospital admission for ≥2 nights "associated with traumatic brain injury on CT"

The researchers did not classify "brief intubations" and single-night admissions for "minor CT findings" as ciTBIs because these outcomes do not typically represent clinically important injuries that must be identified (i.e. patient outcomes would generally be unchanged if these injuries were never diagnosed).

RESULTS

- Table 42.1 lists the six predictive features for ciTBI identified using data from the derivation sample; the strongest predictors of ciTBI in both age groups were an abnormality in mental status or clinical evidence of a skull fracture.
- Table 42.2 divides children into three risk categories using the predictive features.
- In the validation sample, 2 children, both older than 2 years, who did not exhibit any of the 6 predictive features were ultimately found to have ciTBIs; both of these children were injured during sport-related activities, neither wore helmets, both had moderate headaches, and both had large frontal scalp hematomas; neither required neurosurgery.

Table 42.1. PREDICTORS OF CLINICALLY IMPORTANT
TRAUMATIC BRAIN INJURIES

Children <2 Years	Children ≥2 Years
Altered mental status[a]	Altered mental status[a]
Palpable or possibly palpable skull fracture	Clinical signs of basilar skull fracture[c]
Occipital, parietal, or temporal scalp hematoma	Loss of consciousness
	Vomiting
Loss of consciousness ≥5 seconds	Severe mechanism of injury[b]
Severe mechanism of injury[b]	Severe headache
Child not acting normally according to parents	

[a]Defined as a Glasgow Coma Scale of 14 or one of the following: agitation, somonolence, repetitive questioning, or a slow response to verbal communication.
[b]Defined as motor vehicle crash with patient ejection, death of another passenger, or rollover; pedestrian or bicyclist without helmet struck by motorized vehicle; falls >5 feet for children ≥2 years or >3 feet for those <2 years; or head struck by high-impact object.
[c]For example: retro-auricular bruising (Battle's sign), periorbital bruising (raccoon eyes), hematotympanum, or cerebral spinal fluid otorrhea or rhinorrhea.

Table 42.2. PROBABILITY OF CLINICALLY IMPORTANT TRAUMATIC
BRAIN INJURIES BASED ON THE PRESENCE OF PREDICTIVE
FEATURES FOR CHILDREN ≥2 YEARS[a]

Risk Category	Percentage of Children in This Category	Probability of ciTBI
Altered mental status or evidence of a basilar skull fracture	14.0%	4.3%
Any of the four predictive features other than altered mental status or basilar skull fracture	27.7%	0.9%
None of the 6 predictive features	58.3%	<0.05%

[a]The numbers are similar for children <2 years except that the predictive features are different (see Table 42.1). For children <2 years, the highest risk category is "Altered mental status or palpable skull fracture."

Criticisms and Limitations: Emergency departments were carefully selected for participation in this study. In real-world practice, clinicians—particularly those with less experience caring for children—may not be able to safely and effectively follow these prediction rules.

Because children change considerably between early infancy and 2 years of age, perhaps the prediction rule for this age group should be further stratified (e.g., a different rule for children <1 year and children ages 1–2 years).

Other Relevant Studies and Information:

- A follow-up analysis involving children in this study demonstrated that children who were observed in the emergency department for a period of time before a decision was made about obtaining a CT scan were less likely to receive a CT scan.[2]
- Some studies have suggested that there may be as many as 1 case of lethal cancer due to radiation for every 1,000–5,000 head CT scans in children.[3]
- Several other prediction rules for determining when CT scans are indicated in children with head trauma have also been developed.[4,5]
- Comparison of 3 clinical prediction rules and physician judgment found that only the prediction rules described in this chapter and physician judgment identified all ciTBIs in evaluated children.[6]

Summary and Implications: This study derived and validated prediction rules that can accurately identify children at very low risk for ciTBI. The authors suggest that one way these rules could be applied is as follows:

- Children with none of the 6 predictive features are at very low risk (<0.05%) for ciTBI and typically do not require CT scans.
- Children with either of the two highest risk features—altered mental status or evidence of a skull fracture—are at high risk (~4%) and should receive CT scans.
- Children with any of the 4 predictive features other than altered mental status or evidence of a skull fracture have an intermediate risk for ciTBI of approximately 0.9%, and the decision about whether or not to obtain a CT should be individualized based on other factors such as the clinician's judgment, the number of predictive features present, serial evaluations of the patient over time, and the family's preferences.

CLINICAL CASE: DETERMINING WHETHER OR NOT TO OBTAIN A HEAD CT

Case History:

An 18-month-old boy is brought to the emergency department by his parents after he fell off his parent's bed. The bed is approximately 3–4 feet off the ground, and he landed on the side of his head. The boy cried for several minutes after the fall, but he has been acting normally since. He did not lose consciousness after the fall.

On examination, he has a small abrasion over his right cheek, and he has tenderness to palpation over parts of the right parietal region of his scalp. He does not have any scalp hematomas or palpable skull fractures. His neurologic examination is normal.

Based on the results of this study, should you order a CT scan to evaluate this boy for a traumatic brain injury?

Suggested Answer:

The boy in this vignette has 1 of the 6 predictive features for a ciTBI for children <2 years: he had a severe mechanism of injury (fall from a height >3 feet). Based on this study, his risk for a ciTBI is approximately 0.9% (a follow-up analysis estimates the risk for children <2 with a severe mechanism of injury but no other predictive features at 0.3%[7]). The authors of this study recommend that for children in this risk category, the decision about whether or not to obtain a head CT should be individualized based on the clinician's judgment and the family's preference.

As this boy's doctor, you might explain to his parents that the risk of brain injury is low. If you order a head CT scan, there is a small chance that you would detect an important abnormality, but most likely you would not. In addition, the radiation from the CT scan could be harmful. Thus, it would be reasonable either to proceed with the CT scan or to monitor the patient closely and only order a CT scan if the boy's condition worsens. You could recommend one of these two strategies to the parents based on your personal preference; however you should engage the parents to determine their preferences and which approach they are most comfortable with.

References

1. Kuppermann et al. Identification of children at very low risk of clinically-important brain injuries after head trauma: a prospective cohort study. *Lancet.* 2009;374:1160–1170.
2. Nigrovic et al. The effect of observation on cranial computed tomography utilization for children after blunt head trauma. *Pediatrics.* 2011;127(6):1067–1073.
3. Brenner DJ, Hall EJ. Computed tomography—an increasing source of radiation exposure. *N Engl J Med.* 2007;357:2277–2284.
4. Maguire et al. Should a head-injured child receive a head CT scan? A systematic review of clinical prediction rules. *Pediatrics.* 2009;124(1):e145.
5. Pickering et al. Clinical decision rules for children with minor head injury: A systematic review. *Arch Dis Child.* 2011;96(5):414–421.
6. Easter et al. Comparison of PECARN, CATCH, and CHALICE rules for children with minor head injury: A prospective cohort study. *Ann Emerg Med.* 2014;64(2):145–152.
7. Nigrovic et al. Prevalence of clinically important traumatic brain injuries in children with minor blunt head trauma and isolated severe injury mechanisms. *Arch Pediatr Adolesc Med.* 2011 Dec 5.

Oncology

43

Health-Related Quality of Life among Children with Acute Lymphoblastic Leukemia

NINA SHAPIRO

Children with [acute lymphoblastic leukemia] experience very large [health-related quality of life] deficits over the course of treatment: Equivalent to losing approximately 2 months of life in perfect health.

—FURLONG ET AL.[1]

Research Question: What deficits in health-related quality of life (HRQL) exist among children with acute lymphoblastic leukemia (ALL) during active treatment and after treatment, and are there specific disabilities that can be addressed to improve disability without compromising survival?[1]

Funding: Grants from the National Institutes of Health and Garil Fund

Year Study Began: 1995

Year Study Published: 2012

Study Location: 5 centers in the United States and Canada: DFCI/Children's Hospital Boston, Boston, MA; Hôpital Sainte Justine, Montreal, Quebec, Canada; Le Centre Hospitalier de L'Université Laval, Quebec City, Canada;

Maine Children's Cancer Program and Barbara Bush Children's Hospital at Maine Medical Center, Portland, Maine; and McMaster Children's Hospital, Hamilton, Ontario, Canada

Who Was Studied: Children >5 years of age diagnosed with acute lympho-blastic leukemia (ALL) were enrolled either at diagnosis or later, if patients were too young to be eligible at diagnosis. Control groups of similar age and gender distribution were selected from published Canadian sources.

Who Was Excluded: Children <5 years of age as well as children who failed treatment, experienced disease relapses during the posttreatment phase, underwent a bone marrow transplant, or received palliative care were excluded from the study.

How Many Patients: 375

Study Overview: See Figure 43.1 for a summary of the study's design.

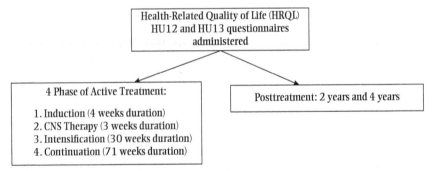

Figure 43.1 Summary of the Study's Design.

Study Intervention: HRQL was measured using HEALTH UTILITIES INDEX© (HUI©) Mark 2 and Mark 3 (HUI2 and HUI3) questionnaires administered to parents, clinicians, and patients themselves if >12 years of age, during the 4 major phases of active treatment and at both 2 and 4 years after treatment. The HUI2 and HUI3 questionnaires collectively assessed sensation, vision, hearing, speech, mobility, ambulation, dexterity, emotion, cognition, self-care, and pain. HRQL scores were used to calculate quality-adjusted life years (QALYs), a metric aggregating both quality and quantity of life.

To assess the effects of different therapy regimens on HRQL, the following treatment randomizations were made:

- Either *E. coli* asparaginase or *Erwinia* L-asparaginase was administered during the induction phase of therapy.
- High-risk patients were given doxorubicin during induction with or without dexrazoxane, a cardioprotectant agent.
- Standard-risk patients received CNS therapy with or without cranial radiation, while high-risk patients received CNS therapy with either hyperfractionated or daily cranial radiation.

Follow-Up: 2 years and 4 years after treatment.

Endpoints: The primary endpoints were HRQL scores throughout the 4 phases of active treatment, HRQL scores at 2 years and 4 years posttreatment, and the difference in HRQL scores between ALL patients and control groups. The authors also evaluated the effects of gender, diagnostic risk group, age at diagnosis, type of asparaginase administered, CNS radiation fractions, and administration of cardioprotectant with radiation on HRQL scores.

RESULTS

- ALL patients experienced a loss of 0.172 QALYs or 63 quality-adjusted life days, equivalent to losing approximately 2 months of life in perfect health, with 86% of the loss during the intensification and continuation phases of active treatment.
- Although differences in HRQL scores between ALL patients and controls were significant at all phases of active treatment ($P < .001$), HRQL scores in ALL patients increased as therapy progressed. HRQL deficits were categorized as "severe" during induction of remission and "moderate" throughout the rest of active treatment. "Mild" deficits, with no significant difference from the general population, were observed in the posttreatment period ($P > .05$). The increase in HRQL scores throughout treatment was mainly due to improvements in the attributes of mobility/ambulation, emotion, self-care, and pain.
- Excess disability rates, defined as rates of HRQL deficit beyond controls, were statistically significant in the HUI2 and HUI3 attributes of mobility, ambulation, dexterity, emotion, self-care, and pain throughout the active treatment period.
- There were no significant effects of gender, diagnostic risk group, age at diagnosis, CNS radiation fractions, and administration of cardioprotectant with radiation on HRQL scores, but it was observed that *E. coli* L-asparaginase administered during the intensification phase was associated with greater morbidity than *Erwinia*

L-asparaginase ($P = .005$ for HUI2 and $P = .007$ for HUI3). However, this result is no longer applicable to current clinical practice because in recent studies, *Erwinia* L-asparaginase was found to be less effective and associated with a higher risk of relapse than *E. coli* L-asparaginase, and therefore is no longer used in treatment protocols.

Criticisms and Limitations:

- The present study does not address HRQL scores for patients less than 5 years of age, after disease relapse, after bone marrow transplantation, or after palliative care.
- Response rates varied throughout the study's course, from a maximum of 84.5% during the continuation phase to a minimum of 38.6% during the second posttreatment phase, which may bias results and limit generalizability.
- The authors intended to measure HRQL scores at 2 years and 4 years posttreatment, but completion rates were below 40% for the 4-year posttreatment assessment. Analysis was therefore limited to the 2-year posttreatment HRQL assessment, and at this phase no statistical differences were found between the HRQL scores of ALL survivors and control groups. Two years may be too short a time for long-term disabilities to be identified, and therefore future study is needed to elucidate the longstanding effects of ALL on quality of life and disability.
- Patient self-reports were only acquired for patients >12 years of age; however, it has been demonstrated that children by the age of 7 or 8 years can provide reliable responses containing valuable subjective information, especially about pain and emotion, that is not available from parental or clinician reports.[3,4]

Other Relevant Studies and Information:

- A study that explored the long-term effects of childhood cancers in adult survivors found that cancer survivors were significantly more likely to have adverse general health, mental health, activity limitations, and functional impairment, compared to their siblings ($P < .001$).[5]
- The population of pediatric cancer survivors is continuing to grow as the cancer survival rate for children and adolescents increases. The overall probability of 5-year survival has increased from <30% in 1960 to 90% at present.[5,6] The National Cancer Institute's Surveillance Epidemiology and End Results program estimates that as of January

2010, there were approximately 379,100 individuals living in the United States who had been diagnosed with cancer during childhood or adolescence, an increase from the 2005 estimate of 328,650 pediatric cancer survivors.[7]

Summary and Implications: Children undergoing treatment for ALL experience large HRQL deficits equivalent to losing 2 months of life in perfect health, especially in the attributes of ambulation/mobility, emotion, and pain. These results identify areas for improvement in current ALL treatment regimens, aiming to reduce disability without compromising relapse rates and survival.

CLINICAL CASE: HEALTH-RELATED QUALITY OF LIFE IN CHILDREN WITH ALL

Case History:

A 9-year-old boy with a new diagnosis of ALL presents to your outpatient clinic as a new patient. He is about to undergo treatment, and his mother wishes to know what to expect regarding the upcoming years, specifically related to his HRQL. What information can you offer this family?

Suggested Answer:

According to the study by Furlong et al., the majority of children who undergo therapy for ALL will have HRQL disability in the areas of mobility/ambulation, dexterity, emotion, self-care, and pain during the treatment periods. However, at 2–4 years posttreatment completion for ALL, most children will have comparable HRQL to those of age-matched children with no prior history of ALL. While longer-term quality of life issues and chronic health issues may ensue, patients in the early years following treatment for ALL have been shown to have HRQL scores similar to those of their peers in the general population.

References

1. Furlong W, Rae C, Feeny D, et al. Health-related quality of life among children with acute lymphoblastic leukemia. *Pediatr Blood Cancer.* 2012;59(4):717–724.
2. Horsman J, Furlong W, Feeny D, Torrance G. The Health Utilities Index (HUI®): concepts, measurement properties and applications. *Health Qual Life Outcomes* 2003;1:54 (electronic journal) http://www.hqlo.com/content/1/1/54.
3. Pickard AS, Topfer LA, Feeny DH. A structured review of studies on health-related quality of life and economic evaluation in pediatric acute lymphoblastic leukemia. *J Natl Cancer Inst Monogr.* 2004;33:102–125. Review.

4. Parsons SK, Barlow SE, Levy SL, Supran SE, Kaplan SH. Health-related quality of life in pediatric bone marrow transplant survivors: according to whom? *Int J Cancer Suppl.* 1999;12:46–51.

5. Hudson MM, Mertens AC, Yasui Y, Hobbie W, Chen H, Gurney JG, Yeazel M, et al. Health status of adult long-term survivors of childhood cancer: a report from the Childhood Cancer Survivor Study. *JAMA.* 2003;290(12):1583–1592.

6. Waters EB, Wake MA, Hesketh KD, Ashley DM, Smibert E. Health-related quality of life of children with acute lymphoblastic leukaemia: comparisons and correlations between parent and clinician reports. *Int J Cancer.* 2003;103(4):514–518.

7. Ries LAG, Smith MA, Gurney JG, et al., eds. *Cancer Incidence and Survival among Children and Adolescents: United States SEER Program 1975–1995.* Bethesda, MD: National Cancer Institute, SEER Program. NIH Pub. No. 99–4649; 1999.

Ophthalmology

44

Treatment of Acute Conjunctivitis in Children

NINA SHAPIRO

Polymyxin B-trimethoprim continues to be an effective treatment for acute conjunctivitis with a clinical response rate that does not differ from moxifloxacin. Use of polymyxin B-trimethoprim for the treatment of conjunctivitis would result in significant cost savings compared with fluoroquinolones.

—WILLIAMS ET AL.[1]

Research Question: Are fluoroquinolones, specifically moxifloxacin, superior to polymyxin B-trimethoprim for the treatment of acute conjunctivitis in children?[1]

Funding: Not listed.

Year Study Began: 2007

Year Study Published: 2013

Study Location: Golisano Children's Hospital Pediatric Ambulatory Clinic and Pittsford Pediatrics in New York.

Who Was Studied: Children 1–18 years of age with a clinical diagnosis of conjunctivitis by the primary physician. Conjunctival swabs for culture were obtained by the study personnel after study enrollment.

Who Was Excluded: Children with suspected allergies, with a recent history of foreign body or trauma to the eye, those who used antibiotics during the previous week or during the study, and those who were non-English speakers were excluded from the study.

How Many Patients: 124

Study Overview: See Figure 44.1 for a summary of the study's design.

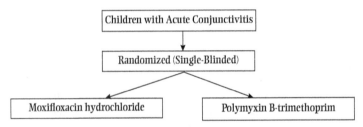

Figure 44.1 Summary of the Study's Design.

Study Intervention: Patients presenting with acute conjunctivitis had bacterial cultures of the affected eye and were randomized to receive therapy with either 0.5% moxifloxacin hydrochloride applied 4 times a day or polymyxin B-trimethoprim applied 3 times a day for 7 days.

Follow-Up: Clinical response was evaluated by phone query 4–6 days after treatment initiation and at a follow-up visit 7–10 days after treatment initiation. At the 7–10 day visit, follow-up conjunctival cultures determined bacteriologic response to therapy.

Endpoints: The primary endpoints of the study were clinical cure rate at 4–6 days and both clinical and bacteriological cure rate at 7–10 days. Clinical cure was defined by complete resolution of all signs and symptoms of conjunctivitis. The specific pathogens isolated from the conjunctival cultures were reported to determine etiology. The MIC90 against *Streptococcus pneumoniae* and *Haemophilus influenzae* were obtained for polymyxin B-trimethoprim and moxifloxacin to determine antibiotic potency.

(MIC90 = Minimal Inhibitory Concentration of a given agent required to inhibit growth of 90% of organisms.)

RESULTS

- There was no significant difference between the groups in clinical cure rate at 4–6 days or 7–10 days. Clinical cure at 4–6 days was 77% for the moxifloxacin group and 72% for those receiving polymyxin B-trimethoprim ($P = 0.59$, noninferiority test with margin 20% $P = 0.04$). At 7–10 days, clinical cure was achieved in 95% of the patients in the moxifloxacin group and in 96% of the patients in the polymyxin B-trimethoprim group (noninferiority test $P \leq 0.01$).
- 65% of patients had a positive bacteriologic culture, and the most commonly isolated pathogens were *H. influenzae, S. pneumoniae,* and *Moraxella catarrhalis.*
- There was no difference in clinical cure rates between patients from whom a pathogen was isolated and those who had a negative culture, regardless of which drug was used.
- Of all the patients who had a positive bacteriologic culture at presentation, there was no significant difference in bacteriologic cure rates between patients receiving moxifloxacin and those receiving polymyxin B-trimethoprim. Bacteriologic cure was seen in 79% of patients who received moxifloxacin and in 61% of patients who received polymyxin B-trimethoprim ($P = 0.52$).
- Moxifloxacin had a much lower MIC90 for both *S. pneumoniae* and *H. influenza* and is therefore considered to be more potent than both polymyxin B and trimethoprim. However, the increased antibiotic potency of moxifloxacin did not impact clinical outcome.

Criticisms and Limitations:

- Although moxifloxacin had a significantly lower MIC90 than polymyxin B-trimethoprim, this difference did not translate to an improved clinical outcome. MIC90 data have been developed to reflect systemic, not topical, treatment. Therefore, the clinical relevance of MIC90 data for topical antibiotic therapy is unknown.
- The absence of a placebo group, along with the observation that no difference in outcome was seen between those patients with

positive initial cultures and those with sterile cultures, raises
the issue as to whether antimicrobial therapy has a role in the
treatment of conjunctivitis.

- Patient compliance was not monitored during the study, so there
  is a possibility that some patients who received follow-up phone
  calls or who came in for follow-up evaluations either did not use
  the drug correctly, or did not use the drug with the prescribed
  dosing.

Other Relevant Studies and Information:

- Acute conjunctivitis is primarily infectious in origin. Most cases
  of conjunctivitis are caused by viruses, but children are more
  likely to acquire conjunctivitis of bacterial origin than viral
  origin.[2] Gigliotti et al. cultured the conjunctivae of 99 children
  with acute conjunctivitis and found that bacteria, namely
  H. influenzae and S. pneumoniae, were responsible for 65% of the
  cases of acute conjunctivitis, while adenoviruses were causative
  in 20% of cases.[3] Weiss et al.'s study of 95 children with acute
  conjunctivitis confirmed that H. influenzae is responsible for most
  cases of bacterial conjunctivitis, followed by S. pneumonia and
  M. catarrhalis.[4]
- Topical antibiotics reduce the duration of symptoms, but more than
  60% of cases of acute bacterial conjunctivitis are self-limited and
  resolve spontaneously within 1–2 weeks.[5]
- Increasing resistance to the most commonly used antibiotics is a
  serious problem; however, all broad-spectrum antibiotics still appear
  to be effective in treating bacterial conjunctivitis.[5]

Summary and Implications: Conjunctivitis is a self-limited infection with
resolution accelerated with topical antibiotics. Contrary to the popular
belief that fluoroquinolones are superior to older antibiotics because of their
increased potency, this study found that topical polymyxin B-trimethoprim
and moxifloxacin were equally effective for the treatment of acute conjunctivitis. Polymyxin B-trimethoprim is significantly less costly than moxifloxacin, and the use of polymyxin B-trimethoprim rather than a fluoroquinolone
for the treatment of conjunctivitis could save more than $300 million per
year based on an estimated 3.7 million annual cases of conjunctivitis in the
United States.[1]

CLINICAL CASE: TREATMENT OF ACUTE CONJUNCTIVITIS

Case History:

A 4-year-old boy is being seen in your office for a 2-day history of right eye discharge, redness, itching, and mild pain. His parents report that he awoke this morning with his eye "sealed shut" with crust. Examination of the eye demonstrates thick, yellow discharge at the lacrimal punctum, conjunctival injection, and mild lid edema. His extraocular mobility and gross visual exam were normal. What is your recommended treatment?

Suggested Answer:

According to the study by Williams et al., polymyxin B-trimethoprim drops, 4 times per day for 7 days, is recommended. While a large number of cases of conjunctivitis are viral in origin, prior studies (Gigliotti et al. 1984) have demonstrated faster cure rate using topical antibiotics than using placebo alone. The current study advocates for polymyxcin B-trimethoprim over moxifloxacin drops. While moxifloxacin was found to have a faster bacterial resolution rate, there was no difference in clinical outcomes between the two treatments. However, there is a significant cost savings (approximately $90/patient) using polymyxin B-trimethoprim over moxifloxacin. Given the high incidence of this disease (approximately 3.7 million visits/year in children <18 years), using polymyxin B-trimethoprim can save up to $300 million per year in health care expenditure.

References

1. Williams L, Malhotra Y, Murante B, et al. A single-blinded randomized clinical trial comparing polymyxin B-trimethoprim and moxifloxacin for treatment of acute conjunctivitis in children. *J Pediatr.* 2013;162(4):857–861.
2. Epling J. Bacterial conjunctivitis. *BMJ Clin Evid.* 2012 Feb 20;2012:0704.
3. Gigliotti F, Williams WT, Hayden FG, et al. Etiology of acute conjunctivitis in children. *J Pediatr.* 1981;98(4):531–536.
4. Weiss A, Brinser JH, Nazar-Stewart V. Acute conjunctivitis in childhood. *J Pediatr.* 1993;122(1):10–14.
5. Azari AA, Barney NP. Conjunctivitis: a systematic review of diagnosis and treatment. *JAMA.* 2013;310(16):1721–1729.
6. Gigliotti F, Hendley JO, Morgan J, Michaels R, Dickens M, Lohr J. Efficacy of topical antibiotic therapy in acute conjunctivitis in children. *J Pediatr.* 1984;104:623–626.

45

Screening for Amblyopia

NINA SHAPIRO

Early treatment is more effective than later treatment for amblyopia, supporting the principle of preschool vision screening.

—WILLIAMS ET AL.[2]

Research Question: How early in life can children with amblyopia be identified, what are the most effective screening methods, and is preschool vision screening warranted for early detection?[1]

Funding: Medical Research Council (United Kingdom), the Wellcome Trust, the UK Department of Health and the Department of the Environment

Year Study Began: 1993

Year Study Published: 2000

Study Location: University of Bristol and University of East Anglia, United Kingdom.

Who Was Studied: Children born during the last 6 months of the Avon Longitudinal Study of Pregnancy and Childhood (ALSPAC), a geographically defined population birth cohort study that includes 14,000 children born between April 1, 1991 and December 31, 1992.

Who Was Excluded: Children born in the first 15 months of the ALSPAC birth period and children whose parents had more than one child in the ALSPAC were excluded.

How Many Patients: 3,490 children; 2,029 children in the intervention group and 1,461 in the control group

Study Overview: See Figure 45.1 for a summary of the study's design.

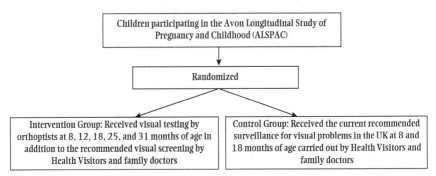

Figure 45.1 Summary of the Study's Design.

Study Intervention: Children in the intervention group received an intensive program of visual assessments by orthoptists at the ages of 8, 12, 18, 25, and 31 months in addition to the current recommended visual screening program in the United Kingdom at 8 and 18 months of age received by the control group. These additional assessments included testing of visual acuity, ocular alignment, stereopsis, motor fusion, and non-cycloplegic photorefraction. Orthoptists are a group of professionals seen more commonly in the United Kingdom and Europe than in the United States. They are trained to examine ocular motility in great detail, and often work closely with optometrists to manage simple childhood vision problems such as strabismus and amblyopia. Children with abnormal results and visual defects were referred to the Hospital Eye Services for further examination.

- Visual acuity was tested using 3 methods: behavior when one eye was occluded (all ages), Cardiff Cards (all ages), and Kay's Pictures (ages 25 and 31 months). Children were referred for further testing if they objected occlusion of one eye more than the other or had Cardiff Cards or Kay Pictures results below normal.
- Ocular alignment was tested using the cover test, and children were referred for suspected strabismus if there was any deviation, latent esophoria, or poorly controlled or large latent exophoria.

- Non-cycloplegic photorefraction was tested using pediatric refractometers at all ages, and data were used to evaluate photorefraction and refractive error as a potential screening tool for amblyopia.

Follow-Up: Follow-up assessments were conducted at 37 months of age, 6 months after the last screening in the intervention group and 19 months after the last screening in the control group, to detect any missed cases of amblyopia or strabismus and to determine the sensitivity of both programs.

Endpoints: The primary endpoints of the study were the number of children referred to the Hospital Eye Services and the number of children subsequently confirmed to have strabismus or amblyopia before 37 months of age. Investigators also determined the sensitivities and specificities of the different vision tests applied at different ages to identify the most effective screening tools.

RESULTS

- A total of 282 children, 147 from the intervention group and 135 from the control group, were referred to the Hospital Eye Services before 37 months of age. 109 children were referred from the final assessment clinic at 37 months of age.
- The cumulative incidence of amblyopia in this study was 2.5%. The intervention group yielded more children with amblyopia than the control group (1.6% vs. 0.5%) before 37 months of age and also detected straight-eyed amblyopia in 0.5% of the population, whereas there were no cases of straight-eyed amblyopia identified in the control group before 37 months of age.
- The control protocol, which is currently the standard program carried out in the United Kingdom, was less sensitive and less specific than the intervention protocol for detecting amblyopia and/or strabismus. Of the children referred to the eye clinic for further evaluation, more children from the intervention group were diagnosed with amblyopia (2.3%) compared with the control group (1.2%), demonstrating the increased sensitivity of the intervention program ($P < 0.01$). The intervention protocol also had a specificity of 95%, while the control protocol had a specificity of 92% with significantly more false positives ($P < 0.01$).
- Even though the intervention program had a higher sensitivity than the control protocol, only 68% of all cases of amblyopia or strabismus could be detected before age 37 months. Sensitivity was highest for

strabismic amblyopia, in which 100% of cases were detected before 37 months, and lowest for straight-eyed amblyopia, most of which could not be identified until age 37 months.

- Cover testing for ocular alignment and visual acuity testing were more than 99% specific at all ages but poorly sensitive until 25 months for ocular alignment and 37 months for visual acuity.
- Photorefraction testing to detect refractive error, on the other hand, when combined with cover testing, was more sensitive but less specific than acuity testing at all ages <37 months. Therefore, photorefraction plus cover testing would have detected more children <37 months old with amblyopia than did cover testing with visual acuity testing but with more false positives. At 37 months, cover testing plus either visual acuity testing or photorefraction are comparable and yield the highest sensitivity and specificity for amblyopia screening.
- Williams et al. conducted a follow-up study that found that the more intensive screening program used in the intervention group was associated with better visual acuity in the amblyopic eye and a decreased prevalence of amblyopia at 7.5 years of age compared with children in the control group. This follow-up data confirm that earlier screening and treatment for amblyopia leads to improved outcome.[2]

Criticisms and Limitations:

- The intervention program used in this study was very intensive and was not designed to be implemented but instead to provide data regarding which screening tools were most efficacious at different ages. Further study is needed to elucidate efficacy of programs that would be feasible to put into practice.
- Attendance at clinics for the intervention program was not optimal, with 69% of patients in the intervention group attending one clinic and 43% attending every clinic, which may have biased results. However, to account for this, all children were included in the analysis regardless of whether or not they had attended the clinics that were offered, which allowed the authors to estimate the effect of being offered the intervention program rather than actually receiving it.

Other Relevant Studies and Information: In the United States, the Maternal and Child Health Bureau and National Eye Institute Task Force on Vision Screening in the Preschool Child produced a report in 2000. This analyzed guidelines for testing including monocular distance acuity and stereopsis screening. They brought forth the need to create standardized statewide guidelines, addressed issues of healthcare professionals' reimbursements, and the cost of amblyopia treatment, both in terms of financial burden and social impact. Implementation of standardized result monitoring was also presented.[3]

The American Academy of Pediatrics, the American Association of Certified Orthoptists, the American Association for Pediatric Ophthalmology and Strabismus, and the American Academy of Ophthalmology issued a Policy Statement regarding routine eye examination in young children by the primary pediatrician. For children between birth and 36 months, routine visual exam should include: (1) ocular history, (2) vision assessment (by fix and follow maneuvers), (3) external inspection of lids and eyes, (4) ocular motility assessment, (5) pupil examination, and (6) red reflex examination.[4]

Summary and Implications: The intervention protocol, consisting of intensive visual screening by orthoptists, was more sensitive and more specific in detecting amblyopia in children <37 months of age than the control protocol currently used in the study population. Since earlier and repeated screening and treatment is associated with improved outcome later in life, this study supports the rationale for additional screening to detect amblyopia earlier in life and preschool vision screening.[1,2] More intensive visual screening in young children is associated with better visual acuity in the amblyopic eye and an overall decreased incidence of amblyopia at age 7.5 years.[2]

CLINICAL CASE: SCREENING FOR AMBLYOPIA IN PRESCHOOL CHILDREN

Case History:
A 12-month-old infant had one assessment 4 months prior to assess visual acuity. It was considered unremarkable at that time. At his 12-month visit, he was noted to have asymmetric ocular alignment. What are your recommendations?

Suggested Answer:
According to Williams et al.[1,2] more detailed evaluation, including visual acuity, ocular alignment, stereopsism motor fusion, and non-cycloplegic photorefraction in young children will better detect children with possible amblyopia and/or strabismus. Referral to a pediatric ophthalmologist or orthoptist is warranted.

References

1. Williams C, Harrad RA, Harvey I, Sparrow JM; ALSPAC Study Team. Screening for amblyopia in preschool children: results of a population-based, randomized controlled trial. ALSPAC Study Team. Avon Longitudinal Study of Pregnancy and Childhood. *Ophthalmic Epidemiol.* 2001;8(5):279–295.
2. Williams C, Northstone K, Harrad RA, Sparrow JM, Harvey I; ALSPAC Study Team. Amblyopia treatment outcomes after screening before or at age 3 years: follow up from randomised trial. *BMJ.* 2002;324(7353):1549.
3. Hartmann EE, Dobson V, Hainline L, et al. Preschool vision screening: Summary of Task Force Report. *Pediatrics.* 2000;106(5):1105–1112.
4. Swanson J, Buckley EG, et al. Policy Statement: Eye examination in infants, children, and young adults by pediatricians. *Pediatrics.* 2003;111(4):902–907.

Orthopedics

46

Differentiation between Septic Arthritis and Transient Synovitis of the Hip in Children

MICHAEL LEVY

The clinical prediction rule for the differentiation between septic arthritis and transient synovitis of the hip in children demonstrated diminished, but nevertheless very good, diagnostic performance in a new patient population.
—KOCHER ET AL.[1]

Research Question: Can a simple clinical prediction rule effectively differentiate septic arthritis versus transient synovitis of the hip?[1]

Funding: None.

Year Study Began: 1997

Year Published: 2004

Study Location: Children's Hospital, Boston, Massachusetts.

Who Was Studied: Children presenting with acute hip pain and a differential diagnosis of transient synovitis or septic arthritis.

Who Was Excluded: Children who had incomplete data available (no joint fluid, peripheral white blood cell count, or blood culture); children who received antibiotics; and children with immunocompromise, renal failure, neonatal sepsis, postoperative hip infection, rheumatologic disease, or Legg-Calve-Perthes disease.

How Many Patients: 154

Study Overview: In a prior study the authors created a clinical prediction rule to differentiate septic arthritis from transient synovitis of the hip (see Table 46.1).[2] This study attempted to validate the rule by prospectively applying it to a new patient cohort.

Table 46.1. COMPONENTS OF CLINICAL PREDICTION RULE

History of fever
Non-weight bearing
Erythrocyte sedimentation rate ≥40 mm/hr
Serum white blood cell count >12,000 cells/mm^3

Follow-Up: An average of 11.8 months (range = 5.9–23.7 months).

Endpoints: True septic arthritis was defined as a positive joint bacterial culture or ≥50,000 white blood cells/mm^3 in the joint fluid with a positive blood culture. Presumed septic arthritis was defined as ≥50,000 cells/mm^3 in joint fluid and negative blood and joint fluid cultures. Transient synovitis was defined as <50,000 cells/mm^3 in joint fluid, resolution of symptoms without antibiotics, and no evidence in the medical record of further disease.

RESULTS

- 51 patients (33%) had septic arthritis (see Table 46.2).
- The area under the receiver operating characteristic curve was 0.86, compared with 0.96 in the original study.
- Radiographic evidence of joint effusion was similar in the transient synovitis group and the septic arthritis group (11% vs. 14%, $P = 0.79$).

Table 46.2. PERFORMANCE OF CLINICAL PREDICTION RULE

Number of Predictors	Probability of Septic Arthritis from Original Study	Distribution of Septic Arthritis in Present Study
0	<0.2%	2.0%
1	3.0%	9.5%
2	40.0%	35.0%
3	93.1%	72.8%
4	99.6%	93.0%

Criticisms and Limitations:

- The prediction rule was developed and validated at one tertiary children's hospital, and may not apply to patients in different regions or in community hospitals.
- Positive predictive value depends on disease prevalence, and will be lower in a population with a lower incidence of septic arthritis.
- C-reactive protein (CRP) was not measured due to institutional limitations.

Other Relevant Studies and Information:

- A retrospective study at a different institution found a predicted probability of septic arthritis of only 59.1% when all four variables were present.[3] That population had a greater proportion of patients with transient synovitis. A study in a smaller general hospital found a predicted probability of 59.9%.[4] These findings reflect that positive predictive value is dependent on disease prevalence.
- A later study added CRP >2.0 mg/dL to the clinical prediction rule and found a probability of septic arthritis of 97.5% with all five variables present.[5] Additional studies have also demonstrated the utility of CRP.[6,7]

Summary and Implications: A simple clinical prediction rule consisting of four variables (history of fever, non-weight bearing, erythrocyte sedimentation rate [ESR], and total white blood cell count [WBC]) can help differentiate between septic arthritis and transient synovitis of the hip. CRP may improve the performance of the rule. The rule can help direct evaluation and management of hip pain, but must be used carefully, and in conjunction with clinical judgment and considering disease prevalence in the population.

CLINICAL CASE: DIFFERENTIATION BETWEEN SEPTIC ARTHRITIS AND TRANSIENT SYNOVITIS

Case History:
You are seeing a 4-year-old girl in the emergency department who complains of acute onset unilateral hip pain. She has not had a fever but is unable to bear any weight. You are concerned for possible septic arthritis of the hip. What further evaluation would you like to do, and how will you manage the patient?

Suggested Answer:
Septic arthritis of the hip can be difficult to differentiate from transient synovitis by the clinical picture alone, and you should seek further objective data. If you obtain a WBC and ESR you will be able to apply the clinical prediction rule. A CRP will also be helpful. If the results of all laboratory tests are normal, the patient has one clinical prediction variable and is unlikely to have septic arthritis. She can likely be managed expectantly with close follow-up. If the results are all elevated, the probability of septic arthritis is as high as 97.5% and the patient will require emergent orthopedic consultation as surgical intervention is likely.

References

1. Kocher MS, Mandiga R, Zurakowski D, Barnewolt C, Kasser JR. Validation of a clinical prediction rule for the differentiation between septic arthritis and transient synovitis of the hip in children. *J Bone Joint Surg Am.* 2004;86-A(8):1629–1635.
2. Kocher MS, Zurakowski D, Kasser JR. Differentiating between septic arthritis and transient synovitis of the hip in children: an evidence-based clinical prediction algorithm. *J Bone Joint Surg Am.* 1999;81(12):1662–1670.
3. Luhmann SJ, Jones A, Schootman M, Gordon JE, Schoenecker PL, Luhmann JD. Differentiation between septic arthritis and transient synovitis of the hip in children with clinical prediction algorithms. *J Bone Joint Surg Am.* 2004;86-A(5): 956–962.
4. Sultan J, Hughes PJ. Septic arthritis or transient synovitis of the hip in children: the value of clinical prediction algorithms. *J Bone Joint Surg Br.* 2010;92(9): 1289–1293.
5. Caird MS, Flynn JM, Leung YL, Millman JE, D'italia JG, Dormans JP. Factors distinguishing septic arthritis from transient synovitis of the hip in children. A prospective study. *J Bone Joint Surg Am.* 2006;88(6):1251–1257.

6. Levine MJ, Mcguire KJ, Mcgowan KL, Flynn JM. Assessment of the test characteristics of C-reactive protein for septic arthritis in children. *J Pediatr Orthop.* 2003;23(3):373–377.
7. Singhal R, Perry DC, Khan FN, et al. The use of CRP within a clinical prediction algorithm for the differentiation of septic arthritis and transient synovitis in children. *J Bone Joint Surg Br.* 2011;93(11):1556–1561.

Pulmonary

47

Steroids for the Treatment of Croup

MICHAEL HOCHMAN, REVISED BY NINA SHAPIRO

Our study shows small but important benefits of dexamethasone treatment for children with mild croup . . . [W]e advocate dexamethasone treatment for essentially all children with croup.

—BJORNSON ET AL.[1]

Research Question: Is dexamethasone effective for the treatment of mild croup?[1]

Sponsor: The Canadian Institutes of Health Research as well as two hospital foundations and a research institute.

Who Was Studied: Children with mild croup, "defined as an onset within the previous 72 hours of a seal-like, barking cough and a score of 2 or less out of 17" on the Westley croup scoring system.[2] The Westley score consists of the sum of points assigned for cyanosis, level of consciousness, air entry, stridor, and retractions.

Who Was Excluded: Children with another cause of stridor, chronic lung disease, asthma, another severe systemic disease, or recent treatment with steroids.

How Many Patients: 720

Study Overview: See Figure 47.1 for a summary of the trial's design.

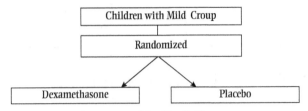

Figure 47.1. Summary of the Trial's Design

Study Intervention: Patients were randomly assigned to receive either a single dose of dexamethasone (suspended in a cherry syrup) 0.6 mg/kg orally (maximum dose 20 mg) or to a placebo syrup.

Follow-Up: 7 days

Endpoints: Primary outcome: return to a medical provider for croup within 7 days of treatment. Secondary outcomes: ongoing symptoms of croup; a cost analysis, which included the cost of dexamethasone, physician costs, hospital costs, and costs to the child's family (e.g. humidifiers and lost productivity); hours of sleep missed by the child; and parental stress resulting from the child's illness.

Data were collected from telephone interviews with parents in the days after treatment as well as from medical records.

RESULTS

- There was a quicker resolution of croup symptoms in the dexamethasone group ($P = 0.003$); however, within 3 days symptoms had completely resolved in >75% of children in both groups (see Table 47.1).
- There was a small but significant reduction in parental stress in the dexamethasone group.

Table 47.1 THE TRIAL'S KEY FINDINGS

Outcome	Dexamethasone Group	Placebo Group	P Value
Return Visits to Medical Provider	7.3%	15.3%	<0.001
Total Costs[a]	$72	$93	0.01
Average Hours of Lost Sleep in First Three Days	2.9	4.2	<0.001

[a]Costs reported in Canadian dollars, which were valued at 70 US cents at the time of the study.

Criticisms and Limitations: Children were recruited for this study from the emergency room; however, many children with mild croup do not visit the emergency room. Children who do not visit the emergency room may have even milder symptoms than those in this study, and therefore may not derive the same benefits from dexamethasone.

Although there were no apparent harmful effects from dexamethasone in this study, the trial was too small to "exclude the possibility of rare adverse events."

Other Relevant Studies and Information: Other trials have demonstrated the benefit of steroids for treating moderate and severe croup[3,4]; however, most children—like those in this study—present with mild symptoms. In cases of moderate to severe croup, whereby children have increased work of breathing with intercostal retractions, the addition of nebulized epinephrine may be warranted.[5]

Summary and Implications: In children with mild croup, a single dose of oral dexamethasone prevents future doctor visits, hastens symptomatic recovery, and lowers overall health care costs.

CLINICAL CASE: STEROIDS FOR THE TREATMENT OF CROUP

Case History:
A 2-year-old previously healthy boy is brought to the emergency room with a 1-day history of mild cold symptoms. Just after bedtime, he was noted by his parents to have a loud, barking cough, with mild stridor. On examination in the emergency room, he has an intermittent barky cough, mild inspiratory stridor, and no cyanosis. His oxygen saturation by pulse oximetry is 97% on room air.

What would be the optimal treatment option?

Suggested Answer:
Based on the Bjornson study, one dose of oral dexamethasone is the best treatment option for this child. One dose of oral dexamethasone for treatment of children with mild croup has been shown to hasten recovery, lessen healthcare visits during the week following symptom onset, reduce parental stress, improve sleep duration, and reduce health care costs.

References

1. Bjornson et al. A randomized trial of a single dose of oral dexamethasone for mild croup. *N Engl J Med.* 2004;351(13):1306–1313.
2. Klassen et al. The croup score as an evaluative instrument in clinical trials. *Arch Pediatr Med.* 1995;149:60.
3. Tibballs et al. Placebo-controlled trial of prednisolone in children intubated for croup. *Lancet.* 1992;340:745–748.
4. Johnson et al. A comparison of nebulized budesonide, intramuscular dexamethasone, and placebo for moderately severe croup. *N Engl J Med.* 1998;339:498–503.
5. Petrocheilou A, Tanou K, Kalampouka E, Malakasioti G, Giannios C, Kaditis AG. Viral croup: diagnosis and treatment algorithm. *Pediatr Pulmonol.* 2014; 49(5):421–429.

Inhaled Corticosteroids for Mild Persistent Asthma

The START Trial

MICHAEL HOCHMAN, REVISED BY NINA SHAPIRO

> Our study has shown that once-daily, low-dose budesonide decreases the risk of severe [asthma] exacerbations . . . in patients with mild persistent asthma. The benefits of this treatment outweigh the small effect on growth in children.
>
> —Pauwels et al.[1]

Research Question: Do inhaled corticosteroids improve outcomes in patients with recent-onset mild persistent asthma?[1]

Funding: The AstraZeneca pharmaceutical company.

Year Study Began: 1996

Year Study Published: 2003

Study Location: 499 sites in 32 countries.

Who Was Studied: Patients 5–66 years old with mild persistent asthma defined as "wheeze, cough, dyspnea, or chest tightening at least once per week, but not as often as daily." Patients were also required to have evidence of reversible airway obstruction on pulmonary function tests (an increase in the forced expiratory volume in 1 second [FEV_1] ≥12% after bronchodilator administration, a decrease in the FEV_1 ≥15% with exercise, or a variation of ≥15% "between the two highest and two lowest peak expiratory flow rates during 14 days") (see Table 48.1).

Table 48.1. ASTHMA CLASSIFICATION IN ADULTS AND CHILDREN ≥5 YEARS

Classification	Days per Week with Symptoms	Nights per Month with Symptoms
Intermittent	≤2	≤2
Mild Persistent[b]	>2	3–4
Moderate Persistent	Daily	≥5
Severe Persistent	Continuous	Frequent

[a]From the National Asthma Education and Prevention Program guidelines.
[b]Most patients in START would be classified as having mild persistent asthma.

Who Was Excluded: Patients with symptoms of asthma for >2 years, those with a history of corticosteroid treatment for more than 30 days, those whose physician felt that corticosteroids should be initiated immediately, those with a prebronchodilator FEV_1 <60% predicted or a postbronchodilator FEV_1 <80% predicted, and those with "another clinically significant disease."

How Many Patients: 7,241

Study Overview: See Figure 48.1 for a summary of the trial's design.

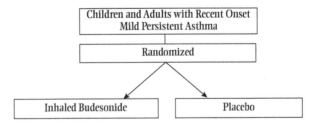

Figure 48.1 Summary of START's Design.

Study Intervention: Patients 11 years of age and older in the inhaled budesonide group received a dose of 400 μg once daily, while those under 11 received a dose of 200 μg once daily. Patients in the placebo group received an inhaled lactose placebo.

Patients in both groups received additional asthma medications, such as inhaled bronchodilators, at the discretion of their physicians. Physicians could prescribe all approved asthma medications including both inhaled and systemic steroids.

Follow-Up: 3 years.

Endpoints: Primary outcome: the time to first severe asthma-related event (an event requiring "admission or emergency treatment for worsening asthma or death due to asthma"). Secondary outcomes: proportion of symptom-free days (based on symptom notebooks kept by patients); the need for additional asthma medications; and the change in prebronchodilator and postbronchodilator FEV_1.

RESULTS

- The mean age of study participants was 24, and 55% were under 18.
- The mean prebronchodilator response of study participants at baseline was 86% predicted, and the mean postbronchodilator response was 96% predicted.
- 23.6% of patients in the placebo group were taking inhaled corticosteroids at the end of the study (recall that in both groups additional asthma medications, including corticosteroids, could be prescribed by each patient's physician for uncontrolled symptoms).
- Patients in the budesonide group experienced fewer asthma-related events than those in the placebo group (see Table 48.2).
- Children ages 5–15 in the budesonide group grew an average of 0.43 cm less per year than children in the control group.

Criticisms and Limitations: The study does not address how inhaled budesonide compares with other inhaled corticosteroids for the treatment of asthma, nor does it provide information about the optimal dose or dosing strategy for inhaled corticosteroids.

Table 48.2. SUMMARY OF START'S KEY FINDINGS

Outcome	Budesonide Group	Placebo Group	*P* Value
Patients with at least one severe asthma-related event[a]	3.5%	6.5%	<0.0001
Proportion of symptom-free days[a]	89%	91%	<0.0001
Patients receiving at least one course of systemic steroids	15%	23%	<0.0001
Change in percent predicted prebronchodilator FEV_1	+3.49%	+1.77%	<0.0001
Change in percent predicted postbronchodilator FEV_1	−1.79%	−2.68%	0.0005

[a]Exact percentages are not reported. These numbers are approximate values from figures.

Other Relevant Studies and Information:

- At the completion of the START trial, all patients—both those in the placebo and budesonide groups—were treated with 2 additional years of open-label budesonide. After a total of 5 years of follow-up, patients in the budesonide group continued to have fewer severe asthma-related events and to require fewer additional asthma medications.[2] Additional analyses of the START trial data have also suggested that budesonide treatment is cost-effective.[3,4]
- Several other studies have also demonstrated the benefit of inhaled corticosteroids in patients with asthma.[5,6]
- The START trial demonstrated a small reduction in height with budesonide. Another study showed that children with asthma who received budesonide had a slightly reduced adult height[7]; however, another analysis suggested that children with asthma who receive long-term treatment with budesonide attain a normal adult height.[8]
- A trial involving preschool children with recurrent wheezing compared daily budesonide with an intermittent use strategy in which children were treated only during episodes of respiratory tract infections. Children in both groups had similar outcomes; however, children in the intermittent dosing group required less medication.[9]

Other studies comparing intermittent use of inhaled corticosteroids with daily use have come to similar conclusions.[10]

Summary and Implications: The START trial showed that daily inhaled budesonide reduces severe asthma exacerbations in children and adults with recent-onset mild persistent asthma. Children 5–15 treated with budesonide had a small but detectable reduction in height compared to children treated with placebo during the 3-year study period. Inhaled corticosteroids are the recommended first-line controller medication for both children and adults with persistent asthma.

CLINICAL CASE: INHALED CORTICOSTEROIDS FOR MILD PERSISTENT ASTHMA

Case History:
An 8-year-old boy with mild asthma since childhood visits your clinic because his asthma has gotten worse over the past month. Instead of using his albuterol inhaler only occasionally, he has recently been using it 3–4 times per week. In addition, he has woken up during the night 3 times in the past month because of his asthma. Upon further questioning, you discover that the boy's parents have been doing construction in their garage over the past month, and their house has been particularly dusty.

Based on the START trial, how should you treat this boy's asthma?

Suggested Answer:
The START trial showed that daily inhaled budesonide reduces severe asthma exacerbations in children and adults with mild persistent asthma. Over the past month, the boy in this vignette has required albuterol more than twice a week and has had 3 nocturnal awakenings per month due to asthma. If these symptoms were to be sustained, this boy would appropriately be classified as having mild persistent asthma.

However, the worsening of this boy's asthma is likely attributable to the dust in his house. You should explain to his parents that the construction in their garage is likely worsening his symptoms, and they should identify ways to reduce their son's exposure to the dust. While it would not be unreasonable to prescribe an inhaled corticosteroid for this boy until the construction is complete, he should not be continued on the steroid indefinitely since such treatment is likely unnecessary and there are adverse effects (e.g., a small but detectable reduction in height, at least in the short term).

References

1. Pauwels RA et al. Early intervention with budesonide in mild persistent asthma: a randomized, double-blind trial. *Lancet*. 2003;361:1071–1076.
2. Busse WW et al. The Inhaled Steroid Treatment As Regular Therapy in Early Asthma (START) study 5-year follow-up: effectiveness of early intervention with budesonide in mild persistent asthma. *J Allergy Clin Immunol*. 2008;121(5):1167.
3. Sullivan SD et al. Cost-effectiveness analysis of early intervention with budesonide in mild persistent asthma. *J Allergy Clin Immunol*. 2003;122(6):1229–1236.
4. Weiss K et al. Cost-effectiveness analysis of early intervention with once-daily budesonide in children with mild persistent asthma: results from the START study. *Pediatr Allergy Immunol*. 2006;17(Suppl 17):21–27.
5. Adams NP et al. Fluticasone vs. placebo for chronic asthma in adults and children. *Cochrane Database Syst Rev*. 2005;(4):CD003135.
6. Adams N et al. Budesonide for chronic asthma in children and adults. *Cochrane Database Syst Rev*. 2001;(4):CD003274.
7. Kelly HW et al. Effect of inhaled glucocorticoids in childhood on adult height. *N Engl J Med*. 2012;367(10):904.
8. Agertoft L, Pederson S. Effect of long-term treatment with inhaled budesonide on adult height in children with asthma. *N Engl J Med*. 2000;343(15):1064–1069.
9. Zeiger RS et al. Daily or intermittent budesonide in preschool children with recurrent wheezing. *N Engl J Med*. 2011;365(21):1990–2001.
10. Papi A et al. Rescue use of beclomethasone and albuterol in a single inhaler for mild asthma. *N Engl J Med*. 2007;356(20):2040–2052.

49

Inhaled Salbutamol (Albuterol) versus Injected Epinephrine in Acute Asthma

NINA SHAPIRO

In view of its lack of adverse effects and noninvasiveness, we recommend nebulized salbutamol delivered by facemask with oxygen, as the drug of choice in children with acute asthma.

—BECKER ET AL.[1]

Research Question: Does nebulized salbutamol (albuterol), a selective beta-2 agonist, have equal or better efficacy in the treatment of acute asthma in children when compared with injected epinephrine?[1]

Funding: Children's Hospital of Winnipeg Research Foundation.

Year Study Began: 1981

Year Study Published: 1983

Study Location: Children's Hospital of Winnipeg, Manitoba, Canada.

Who Was Studied: Children 6–17 years of age who had previously documented reversible airway obstruction by pulmonary function testing, presenting with acute asthma to the emergency department.

Who Was Excluded: Children who had received treatment for an acute episode of asthma within the last 2 hours.

How Many Patients: 40

Study Overview: See Figure 49.1 for a summary of the study's design.

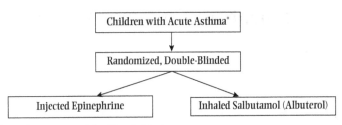

Figure 49.1 Summary of the Trial's Design.
*Severity measured using the Pulmonary Index, which included clinical evidence of elevated respiratory rate, wheezing, altered inspiratory-expiratory ratio, and use of accessory respiratory muscles.

Study Intervention: Children who presented to the emergency room with acute asthma were either given salbutamol (0.5% solution, 0.02 ml/kg, maximum 1 mL) administered by facemask and nebulizer or epinephrine (1:1000 solution, 0.01 mL/kg, maximum 0.4 mL) subcutaneously. In this double-blind study, 20 children were randomly assigned to each study group, and each child received paired solutions for injection and inhalation, one consisting of active drug and the other of saline. Both groups received 30% oxygen via face mask during the intervention. Forced vital capacity (FVC), forced expiratory volume in 1 second (FEV_1), and forced expiratory flow from 25%–75% of the vital capacity ($FEF_{25\%-75\%}$) were measured prior to intervention. Patients remained on room air for 10 minutes before arterial blood was obtained for measurement of blood gases.

Follow-Up: Vital signs and spirometric data were collected at 15 and 30 minutes posttreatment. If necessary, another dose of the prescribed treatment was given at 30 minutes with additional data collection at 45 and 60 minutes after the initial dose. Blood gas samples were obtained 30 minutes after drug administration and after oxygen had been discontinued for 10 minutes.

Endpoints:

- Spirometric data: FEV_1, FVC, $FEF_{25\%-75\%}$, ratio of FEV_1 to FVC (FEV_1/FVC)

- Vital signs: systolic and diastolic blood pressure, pulse, respiratory rate, heart rate
- Blood gases: PaO_2, $PaCO_2$
- Repeat treatment, return to emergency room, subsequent admissions, and total number of admissions within 7 days

RESULTS

- There were no significant differences $(P > .05)$ observed between the groups in pulmonary index, FEV_1, FVC, $FEF_{25\%-75\%}$, FEV_1/FVC, PaO_2, systolic and diastolic blood pressure, respiratory rate, and heart rate.
- In both groups, there was significant improvement in FVC, FEV_1, and $FEF_{25\%-75\%}$. Improvement in FEV_1/FVC was significant in both groups at 15 minutes, but significant improvement in the salbutamol group was only seen at 15 minutes and not thereafter.
- After administration of epinephrine, a significant decrease in diastolic blood pressure and an increase in systolic pressure were seen, while there was no significant change after salbutamol administration.
- No significant change in heart rate was observed in the group given epinephrine, whereas a significant increase in heart rate was seen after salbutamol administration.
- Adverse effects such as nausea, vomiting, tremor, headache, palpitations, excitement, and pallor were seen in 10 out of the 20 children receiving epinephrine, while no adverse effect were seen in those given salbutamol.
- No significant difference in repeat treatment, admission, return to emergency room, or readmission was found between the groups.

Criticisms and Limitations: This paper did not address the possibility of giving multiple successive lower doses of drug versus a single dose to decrease adverse effects. Although some of the patients involved in the study were given corticosteroids upon discharge, the authors did not expand upon on the role of corticosteroids at presentation with an acute asthma exacerbation.

Other Relevant Studies and Information:

- Zorc et al. (1999) found in a meta-analysis of 9 studies that addition of multiple doses of ipratropium in addition to an inhaled beta agonist was beneficial for treatment of children with acute asthma in the emergency department, reducing both duration of treatment times and the number of albuterol doses administered.[2]

- Edmonds et al. conclude that systemic corticosteroids should be given to all patients with acute asthma presenting to the emergency department, and inhaled corticosteroids can be considered in addition to systemic corticosteroid treatment, since they have been shown to decrease hospital admissions compared to placebo.[3]
- Kling et al. determined that inhaled bronchodilators remain the first-line treatment of acute asthma exacerbations. In patients who do not respond to multiple doses of inhaled bronchodilators, nebulized ipratropium bromide should be added. They also recommend oral corticosteroids to prevent relapse of acute symptoms.[4]

Summary and Implications: Among children presenting in the emergency room with acute asthma, there was no significant difference in early efficacy between inhaled salbutamol and subcutaneously injected epinephrine; however, epinephrine injection resulted in significantly more adverse effects and was more invasive. Because of this and subsequent studies, inhaled beta agonists—rather than injected epinephrine—are now recommended as first line therapy for children with acute asthma exacerbations.

CLINICAL CASE: ACUTE ASTHMA EXACERBATION IN CHILDREN

Case History:

An 8-year-old boy with a prior history of asthma presents to the emergency room with a 3-hour history of progressively worsening tachypnea, wheezing, and intercostal retractions. He had not had active asthma-like symptoms for several months, so was not taking any medications at home.

Based on the results of this trial, how would you treat this child?

Suggested Answer:

This trial found that early use of salbutamol (albuterol) within the first few hours of asthma exacerbation lead to effective improvement in pulmonary function, without any notable side effects or adverse events. It is considered to be as effective, and less invasive, with fewer side effects in treating asthma exacerbations than previously recommended epinephrine injection.

References

1. Becker AB, Nelson NA, Simons FE. Inhaled salbutamol (albuterol) vs injected epinephrine in the treatment of acute asthma in children. *J Pediatr.* 1983;102(3):465–469.
2. Zorc JJ, Pusic MV, Ogborn CJ, Lebet R, Duggan AK. Ipratropium bromide added to asthma treatment in the pediatric emergency department. *Pediatrics.* 1999;103(4 Pt 1):748–752.
3. Edmonds ML, Milan SJ, Camargo CA Jr, Pollack CV, Rowe BH. Early use of inhaled corticosteroids in the emergency department treatment of acute asthma. *Cochrane Database Syst Rev.* 2012;12.
4. Kling S, Zar HJ, Levin ME, Green RJ, Jeena PM, Risenga SM, et al. Guideline for the management of Acute Asthma in Children: 2013 update. *S Afr Med J.* 2013;103(3):199–207.

50

Long-term Inhaled Hypertonic Saline for Cystic Fibrosis

JEREMIAH DAVIS

Long-term treatment with hypertonic saline improved lung function, reduced the frequency of exacerbations, and reduced absenteeism in both children and adults.

—ELKINS ET AL.[1]

Research Question: Does long-term inhaled hypertonic saline improve lung function and reduce pulmonary exacerbations in patients with cystic fibrosis?[1]

Funding: US Cystic Fibrosis Foundation, National Health & Medical Research Council of Australia, and the Australian Cystic Fibrosis Research Trust.

Year Study Began: 2000

Year Study Published: 2006

Study Location: 16 adult and pediatric hospitals in Australia.

Who Was Studied: Cystic fibrosis (CF) patients ≥6 years of age whose screening forced expiratory volume in 1 second (FEV_1) was within 10% of their personal best as measured in the last 6 months, and was ≥40% of the predicted value based on age, gender, and height.

Who Was Excluded: Patients whose lung function tests did not meet the above criteria; those who had used hypertonic saline or needed additional antibiotics within 2 weeks of the study start; additionally, pregnant patients or those breastfeeding, cigarette smokers, and those with colonization by *Burkholderia cepacia* species were excluded.

How Many Patients: 164

Study Overview: See Figure 50.1 for a summary of the trial's design.

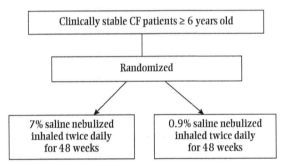

Figure 50.1 Summary of the Trial's Design.

Study Intervention: Patients assigned to the study group inhaled 4 mL of nebulized hypertonic (7%) saline twice daily, preceded by an albuterol bronchodilator. Control patients followed the same procedures except that the saline was isotonic (0.9%) saline. 0.25 mg/mL of quinine sulfate was added to either preparation to disguise taste differences.

Follow-Up: Participants underwent evaluations at 4, 12, 24, and 36 weeks, as well as 2 final visits (within 1 week of each other) at the 48-week end point. Clinical evaluation, sputum sample collection, spirometry, and quality of life questionnaires were collected at each evaluation visit. Weekly cards documenting symptoms were filled out by participants, and pulmonary exacerbations were tracked using changes in signs or symptoms whether or not antibiotics were initiated.

Endpoints: Primary outcome: linear rate of change in lung function compared to baseline. Secondary outcomes: absolute difference in lung function compared to baseline, quality of life survey results, sputum concentration of cytokines and microbiologic character, and number of exacerbations and/or hospitalizations.

RESULTS

- Baseline characteristics between hypertonic and normal saline groups were similar.
- For the primary endpoint (see Table 50.1), a model that incorporated FEV_1, forced vital capacity (FVC), and forced expiratory flow at 25%–75% of the FVC ($FEF_{25\%-75\%}$) did not demonstrate a significant difference in the linear slope of lung function between control and experimental groups ($P = 0.79$).
- Absolute changes in FEV_1 and FVC increased during the initial 4-week study period for hypertonic saline recipients and thereafter plateaued, resulting in a consistent difference for the remainder of the study (Table 50.1); the absolute level of difference in FVC also differed depending on age, with adults ($\geq$18 years) seeing a mean 175 mL higher value (95% CI 56 to 294, $P = 0.004$) among hypertonic saline patients, whereas children (<18 years) saw no significant change (1 mL higher in control group, 95% CI –72 to 70, $P = 0.98$).
- Fewer pulmonary exacerbations needing IV antibiotics occurred among hypertonic saline recipients (0.39 vs. 0.89, mean difference 0.50, 95% CI 0.14 to 0.86, $P = 0.02$), as well as fewer mean number of days of exacerbations and longer periods free of exacerbation.
- When exacerbations were defined by patient symptoms alone, a similar significant difference was noted. The mean number of exacerbations for control subjects (2.74 events/patient) were significantly higher than among hypertonic saline recipients (1.32 events/subject) (mean difference 1.42, 95% CI 0.86 to 1.99, $P < 0.001$).
- These fewer exacerbations resulted in fewer days absent from school or work or inhibiting normal activities, but did not lead to fewer unscheduled hospital visits or stays; no difference in weight or body mass index was noted.
- Cytokine concentrations and microbiologic character were not significantly affected; coliform bacteria were acquired more often in the control group.
- While adverse drug reactions due to the hypertonic saline were more common than with normal saline (14 vs. 1, $P = 0.01$), overall adverse events were significantly lower in the hypertonic group (2.89 vs. 5.17 per 336 days, $P < 0.001$).

Table 50.1. SUMMARY OF THE TRIAL'S KEY FINDINGS

Outcome	FEV$_1$	FVC	FEF$_{25\%-75\%}$	P
Difference between hypertonic saline and control groups in linear rate of change in mL/ week (from 0–48 weeks)[a]	0.3 (–1.3, 1.8)	0.5 (–1.3, 2.3)	–1.5 (–4.2, 1.2)	0.79[b]
Absolute difference between hypertonic saline and control groups in lung function in mL (from week 4–48)[a]	68 (3, 132)	82 (12, 153)	39 (–67, 146)	0.03[b]

[a]Positive values indicate a benefit from hypertonic saline treatment; parentheses indicate 95% confidence intervals.
[b]Result of a single model incorporating all three lung function measurements.

Criticisms and Limitations: Compliance with treatment was similar between both groups (63% in controls, 64% in hypertonic), and while this level is likely reflective of real-world challenges in implementation, it is possible that the benefits of hypertonic saline would have been more pronounced if compliance had been better. There were intriguing differences between those younger than 18 years and adults; thus stratification of the participants by age or perhaps by baseline lung function might have led to insights regarding hypertonic saline's impact at various ages.

Other Relevant Studies and Information:

- Several previous studies examined the short-term effects of hypertonic saline in CF patients; 2 case series published by Robinson et al. demonstrated improved mucociliary clearance with the use of hypertonic saline[2,3]; this was corroborated by improvements in lung function noted by Donaldson et al.[4] and reviewed by the Cochrane Database.[5]
- After publication, use increased in pediatric CF populations and studies focused on safety and tolerability in those even younger than Elkins' participants.[6-8]
- A randomized controlled trial in children <6 years of age with hypertonic saline failed to reduce pulmonary exacerbations or show significant difference in pulmonary function testing.[9]

- While practices differ at various institutions, Cystic Fibrosis Foundation guidelines and general consensus recommend offering inhaled hypertonic saline therapy to patients >6 years of age.[10]

Summary and Implications: This study was the first to evaluate long-term effects of hypertonic saline on the lung function of patients with CF. No difference was noted in the linear slope of lung function during the study period, but there were significant differences noted in absolute lung function, number and length of pulmonary exacerbations, and missed school, work, or activities—all favoring hypertonic saline in patients >6 years of age. Hypertonic saline provides a safe and inexpensive treatment option for reducing CF exacerbations and improving quality of life measures for CF patients.

CLINICAL CASE: REDUCING PULMONARY EXACERBATIONS IN CF PATIENTS

Case History:

A new patient transfers to your primary care clinic from out of state. During the intake visit you note the 9-year-old girl has cystic fibrosis that was diagnosed in infancy. The family is relocating to your town to be closer to a regional pediatric CF center since she "has been in and out of the hospital too many times" over the past few months. On reviewing her home CF regimen you note that she is not receiving hypertonic saline therapy. When you ask if the family has ever used this treatment the parents respond no, and ask you if it's safe to use in children.

What is the best response to their inquiry?

Suggested Answer:

Elkins et al. demonstrated a beneficial effect to routine, long-term hypertonic saline for children as young as 6 years old. In fact, the treatment had a notable effect on pulmonary exacerbations—which this patient is particularly struggling with. The routine use of hypertonic saline has not been shown to be beneficial in children <6 years over a similar 48-week period, but this patient is old enough that the family should ask their new pulmonologists to consider adding hypertonic saline to her daily regimen.

References

1. Elkins MR et al. A controlled trial of long-term inhaled hypertonic saline in patients with cystic fibrosis. *N Eng J Med.* 2006;354(3):229–240.
2. Robinson M et al. Effect of hypertonic saline, amiloride, and cough on mucociliary clearance in patients with cystic fibrosis. *Am J Respir Crit Care Med.* 1996;153(5):1503–1509.
3. Robinson M et al. Effect of increasing doses of hypertonic saline on mucociliary clearance in patients with cystic fibrosis. *Thorax.* 1997;52(10):900–903.
4. Donaldson S et al. Mucus clearance and lung function in cystic fibrosis with hypertonic saline. *N Engl J Med.* 2006;354(3):241–250.
5. Wark P, McDonald VM. Nebulised hypertonic saline for cystic fibrosis. *Cochrane Database Syst Rev.* 2009:CD001506.
6. Rosenfeld M et al. Inhaled hypertonic saline in infants and toddlers with cystic fibrosis: short-term tolerability, adherence, and safety. *Pediatr Pulmonol.* 2011; 46:666–671.
7. Dellon EP et al. Safety and tolerability of inhaled hypertonic saline in young children with cystic fibrosis. *Pediatr Pulmonol.* 2008; 43:1100–1106.
8. Subbarao P et al. Pilot study of safety and tolerability of inhaled hypertonic saline in infants with cystic fibrosis. *Pediatr Pulmonol.* 2007;42:471–476.
9. Rosenfeld M et al. Inhaled hypertonic saline in infants and children less than six years of age with cystic fibrosis: the ISIS randomized trial. *JAMA.* 2012;306(21):2269–2277.
10. Flume PA et al. Cystic fibrosis pulmonary guidelines: chronic medications for maintenance of lung health. *Am J Respir Crit Care Med.* 2007;176(10): 957–969.

Index

References to notes, tables, figures and boxes are denoted by an italicized *n, t, f,* and *b*